Live Well, Age Better

An Australian Doctor's Practical Guide to a Longer, Healthier Life

Dr Mark Lewis

The information in this book is intended as general health education and does not constitute medical advice. Always consult a qualified healthcare professional before making changes to your health management.

ISBN 978-1-7646275-0-4 (Paperback — Amazon KDP)

ISBN 978-1-7646275-1-1 (Paperback — IngramSpark)

ISBN 978-1-7646275-2-8 (Ebook)

First published 2025

Printed in Australia

Introduction

Why Healthspan Matters More Than Lifespan

A Doctor's Honest Admission

I have spent a career spanning pharmacy and medicine working in healthcare — as a pharmacist and as a doctor — and across that time I have seen the full arc of what illness does to a life. I have worked at the sharp end of emergency medicine, where people arrive at their most vulnerable, and I have spent years in integrative and longevity medicine, trying to understand what brought them there in the first place. And I'll be honest with you: for a long time, the system I worked within was focused on treating the consequences of ageing rather than addressing its causes.

Emergency medicine is extraordinary work — urgent, life-saving, and deeply meaningful. But it is, by its very nature, a system that waits for things to go wrong. You arrive broken, and we try to fix you. Whether I was dispensing medications as a pharmacist or managing acute presentations as an emergency doctor, I kept arriving at the same uncomfortable question: what could we have done ten or twenty years ago to keep you from arriving here at all?

That question changed the direction of my career. It also changed how I think about my own health, my patients' health, and ultimately, what I believe medicine should be doing much more of.

This book is the result of that shift in thinking. It is not a book about extreme biohacking, cold plunge obsessions, or a supplement stack that costs more than your mortgage. It is not written for elite athletes or Silicon Valley executives trying to live to 150. It is written for you — an ordinary Australian in your forties, fifties, or sixties who wants to feel well, stay strong, and enjoy a full life for as long as possible.

That is what healthspan means. And in Australia right now, we have a serious problem with it.

We Are Living Longer — But Not Necessarily Better

Australia is one of the longest-lived nations on Earth. According to the Australian Bureau of Statistics, life expectancy at birth is now **81.1 years for males and 85.1 years for females** — figures that would have seemed extraordinary to our grandparents' generation. By global standards, we are doing remarkably well.

But here is the part that does not make the headlines: we are not spending all of those years in good health. Research published in the Journal of the American Medical Association found that Australia has one of the largest gaps between lifespan and healthspan of any nation in the world — a gap of more than twelve years. That means the average Australian can expect to spend over a decade of their life living with significant illness, disability, or chronic disease.

Put another way: we have become very good at keeping people alive. We have not been nearly as good at keeping them well.

"Australia ranks among the world's longest-lived nations — yet the average Australian spends more than twelve years of their life in poor health."

Data from the Australian Institute of Health and Welfare tells a similar story. For males born in 2024, health-adjusted life expectancy — the number of years lived in full health — is 71.7 years. For females, it is 73.8 years. That leaves more than nine years for men, and over eleven years for women, spent managing the consequences of chronic disease, disability, or significant health decline.

The leading causes of this lost healthy time are conditions that are, in large part, preventable: cardiovascular disease, type 2 diabetes, dementia, musculoskeletal disorders, and depression. These are not random acts of biology. They are deeply influenced by how we eat, how we move, how we sleep, how we manage stress — and, critically, how early we start paying attention to all of the above.

This is not a counsel of despair. It is, in fact, one of the most empowering facts in modern medicine. The science tells us that the majority of what determines how well we age is within our influence — not our genes, not our luck, and not our postcode. And the best time to start is now, wherever you are.

Lifespan vs Healthspan: Why the Distinction Matters

If you ask most people what they want from a long life, they do not say 'more years.' They say things like: 'I want to be able to play with my grandchildren.' 'I want to travel while I can still enjoy it.' 'I want to stay sharp, stay independent, and not be a burden to anyone.' 'I want the last chapter of my life to look something like the middle ones.'

What they are describing, without necessarily knowing the word for it, is healthspan.

Healthspan is the number of years you live in good health — free from serious chronic disease, significant disability, and the kind of cognitive or physical decline that limits your ability to fully participate in your own life. It is distinct from lifespan, which simply measures how long you live, regardless of quality.

Modern medicine has been extraordinarily successful at extending lifespan. Antibiotics, vaccines, surgical advances, and intensive care have transformed what it means to survive illness. But in doing so, we have created a new challenge: a large population of people living longer, but living those extra years with chronic conditions that erode quality of life.

The goal of this book is to help close that gap. Not by promising you a magic bullet, but by giving you the evidence-based knowledge — translated into practical, everyday language — to make meaningful changes to how you age. Small, consistent actions, applied over years, can produce remarkable results. The science is clear on this. The challenge is simply knowing where to start.

Why an Australian Perspective Matters

The longevity space has exploded in recent years. Books, podcasts, YouTube channels, and social media accounts — many of them excellent — offer detailed guidance on how to live longer and better. If you have read Peter Attia's Outlive, listened to Andrew Huberman, or dipped into David Sinclair's work on ageing, you have had a taste of what cutting-edge longevity science looks like.

But much of this content is American. And while the underlying biology is universal, the practical application — the food environment, the healthcare system, the tests you can access, the culture around ageing — is not. When a US-based author recommends a specific blood panel, it may not be Medicare-rebatable in Australia. When they discuss particular medications or supplements, Australian availability and regulatory frameworks differ. When they frame exercise or dietary advice, they are not speaking to someone whose nearest GP bulk bills and whose specialist waitlist is six months long.

This book is written with Australia in mind. The practical advice is grounded in what is accessible, affordable, and achievable within the Australian healthcare context. The references to testing, providers, and resources are relevant to where you live. And the voice — I hope — feels like a conversation with your doctor, not a lecture from a laboratory.

I have also tried to bridge two worlds that are too often kept separate: mainstream medicine and integrative medicine. Both have a great deal to offer, and both have limitations. The best outcomes I have seen in my patients come from combining the rigour of evidence-based medicine with the broader lens of integrative practice — looking at the whole person, not just the pathology.

What This Book Is — and What It Is Not

Before we go any further, let me be direct about what you will find here.

This book is not a diet book. You will not find a meal plan, a macronutrient prescription, or a list of foods to eliminate. What you will find is an honest, evidence-based look at the nutritional patterns most consistently associated with long-term health — and a framework for finding an approach that works for your life.

This book is not a fitness manual. I am not going to tell you that you need to run marathons or deadlift twice your bodyweight. What I will tell you is that movement is one of the most powerful medicines available to us, and that even modest, consistent physical activity produces substantial benefits for healthspan.

This book is not a supplement catalogue. While we will explore some emerging therapies — including peptides, NAD+ precursors, and other interventions gaining traction in the longevity space — I will always lead with lifestyle, because that is where the evidence is strongest.

What this book is: a practical, evidence-based companion for anyone who wants to take their long-term health seriously. It is structured to give you both understanding and action — because knowing the science matters, but only if it translates into something you can actually do.

How to Use This Book

Live Well, Age Better is organised into four parts. The first part lays the scientific foundation — explaining how and why we age, and why our chronological birthday is far less important than our biological one. The second part covers the five foundational pillars of healthspan: sleep, movement, nutrition, stress, and connection. These are the non-negotiables. Get these right, and you will have done more for your longevity than any supplement or therapy can offer.

The third part goes deeper into specific areas: hormonal health, the gut-longevity axis, metabolic health, and emerging therapies. This is where the integrative medicine perspective comes into its own, and where some of the most exciting recent science lives. The fourth part brings it all together, helping you build a personalised healthspan plan that is realistic for your life, your budget, and your starting point.

You do not need to read this book in order, though I recommend it for the first pass. Each chapter is written to stand alone, so if sleep is your burning issue, start there. If your gut is playing up, skip ahead. Use this book the way you would use a good GP — ask it the questions that matter most to you right now.

At the end of each section, you will find a practical summary — the key actions to take, in plain language, with no fluff.

A Word on Hope — and Honesty

I want to close this introduction with something that might surprise you coming from a doctor: I am genuinely optimistic about what is possible for your health.

Not naively optimistic. I have sat with patients who have left it too late, who have spent decades ignoring the signals their bodies were sending, and who arrived in my clinic carrying the accumulated weight of decades of unhelpful habits. That is a hard conversation. But even then — even in those cases — it is rarely too late to make meaningful change.

The science of ageing has transformed in the past twenty years. We now understand, at a level of detail that was unimaginable a generation ago, the biological mechanisms that drive ageing — and the levers we can pull to slow them down. We have strong evidence that the choices you make in your forties and fifties can dramatically shape your seventies and eighties. And we are beginning to develop tools — pharmacological, technological, and lifestyle-based — that may extend not just how long we live, but how well we live those years.

None of this requires perfection. It requires consistency, curiosity, and a willingness to take your own health as seriously as you take everything else you care about.

You picked up this book. That is a good start. Let's get into it.

References

Australian Bureau of Statistics. (2024). Life expectancy, 2022–2024. ABS. https://www.abs.gov.au/statistics/people/population/life-expectancy/latest-release

Australian Institute of Health and Welfare. (2024). Deaths in Australia: Life expectancy. AIHW. https://www.aihw.gov.au/reports/life-expectancy-deaths/deaths-in-australia/contents/life-expectancy

Djordjevic, M., et al. (2024). Global healthspan-lifespan gaps among 183 World Health Organization member states. JAMA Network Open, 7(12), e2451614. https://pmc.ncbi.nlm.nih.gov/articles/PMC11635540/

Centre for Healthy Brain Ageing (CHeBA), UNSW Sydney. (2021). Healthy life expectancy across Australia on the rise as latest global disease estimates revealed. https://www.cheba.unsw.edu.au

Caulfield, T., et al. (2023). Australians are living and working longer — but not necessarily healthier.

University of Wollongong. https://www.uow.edu.au/media/2023

GBD 2019 Diseases and Injuries Collaborators. (2020). Global burden of 369 diseases and injuries in 204 countries and territories, 1990–2019. The Lancet, 396(10258), 1204–1222.

Attia, P. (2023). Outlive: The science and art of longevity. Harmony Books.

Lopez-Otin, C., et al. (2023). Hallmarks of aging: An expanding universe. Cell, 186(2), 243–278.

Australian Institute of Health and Welfare. (2024). Australian Burden of Disease Study 2024: Health-adjusted life expectancy. AIHW.

Chapter One

The Hallmarks of Ageing

---

*What is actually happening inside your
body — and why it matters*

Picture a brand-new car rolling off the production line. Every component is precisely engineered, every system running smoothly. For a while, very little maintenance is needed. But time passes. Rubber seals begin to harden. Fluids degrade. Metal components fatigue under the stress of repeated use. Some parts fail quietly and are compensated for by others. Eventually, a threshold is crossed — and what had been seamless performance becomes unreliable, then fragile, then finally, it stops altogether.

Your body is infinitely more complex and resilient than any machine — but it ages by a surprisingly similar principle. Over time, damage accumulates at the cellular level. Repair systems that once ran efficiently begin to fall behind. Tissues that were once renewed with precision start to show errors. And the downstream consequences of this accumulating cellular damage are the chronic diseases — heart disease, cancer, dementia, type 2 diabetes, osteoporosis — that define poor health in later life.

For most of human history, we understood ageing as something that simply happened. A clock wound down, a candle burned out. But in the past three decades, science has revealed something far more useful: ageing is not a single process. It is the sum of specific, identifiable biological mechanisms — mechanisms that we can study, measure, and in many cases, meaningfully influence.

In 2013, a team of leading researchers published what has become one of the most cited papers in the history of biology — a framework they called the Hallmarks of Ageing. The paper, published in the journal Cell and authored by Carlos López-Otín and colleagues, identified nine core biological processes that drive ageing at the cellular level. A decade later, in 2023, the same team returned with an updated framework, expanding the list to twelve hallmarks as the science had advanced. This framework is now the foundation of virtually all serious longevity research worldwide.

You do not need to memorise any of this. But understanding the broad strokes of what these hallmarks are — and crucially, which ones you can influence through your daily choices — is one of the most empowering things you can take from this book. Because once you understand what drives ageing at the cellular level, the advice in the chapters that follow stops feeling like a list of rules and starts making genuine sense.

What Makes Something a Hallmark of Ageing?

The researchers who developed this framework set three criteria for something to qualify as a hallmark of ageing. First, it must appear and worsen as a normal part of getting older. Second, deliberately accelerating it should speed up ageing. And third — most importantly for our purposes — slowing it down or reversing it should extend healthy lifespan.

That third criterion is the key one. The hallmarks are not just a list of things that go wrong with age. They are a map of the biological levers that, when pulled in the right direction, can meaningfully change how well and how long you live.

The twelve hallmarks fall into three broad categories. The first group — what the researchers call the primary hallmarks — are the root causes, the original sources of damage that accumulate over time. The second group are the compensatory hallmarks: biological responses that initially try to repair the damage, but which eventually become problems themselves. The third group are the integrative hallmarks — the downstream consequences that arise when the first two groups tip out of balance and begin to affect whole tissues and organ systems.

Let's walk through each one. I'll keep it practical — what it is, why it matters, and what you can do about it.

The Primary Hallmarks: Where Ageing Begins

1. Genomic Instability

Every cell in your body contains roughly three billion base pairs of DNA — the complete instruction manual for how you work. Every time a cell divides, that entire manual must be copied with extraordinary precision. And every day, your DNA is subjected to thousands of small acts of damage: ultraviolet radiation, oxidative stress, errors in copying, environmental toxins.

Your body has sophisticated repair systems to address this damage — and for most of your life, they do an impressive job. But repair is never perfect, and over time, small errors accumulate. This accumulated genomic instability is considered the primary driver of ageing, and it underlies the increased risk of cancer, cellular malfunction, and tissue decline that comes with age.

What you can do: Chronic inflammation, smoking, excess alcohol, and UV exposure all accelerate DNA damage. Conversely, antioxidant-rich foods, regular exercise, and adequate sleep support your body's DNA repair mechanisms. These are not small effects — they are significant.

2. Telomere Attrition

Telomeres are the protective caps at the ends of your chromosomes — imagine the plastic tips on the end of a shoelace, preventing the lace from fraying. Each time a cell divides, the telomeres get a little shorter. When they become critically short, the cell can no longer divide safely and enters a state called senescence (more on this shortly) or is destroyed altogether.

Telomere length is now widely regarded as one of the best available markers of biological age. People with longer telomeres for their age tend to be healthier and live longer. And critically, the rate at which your telomeres shorten is not fixed — it is influenced significantly by lifestyle.

Research published in The Lancet Oncology found that comprehensive lifestyle changes — including a plant-based diet, moderate exercise, stress management, and social connection — were associated with a significant increase in telomere length over five years. This was the first controlled trial to show that any intervention could actually lengthen telomeres in humans (Ornish et al., 2013).

A systematic review and meta-analysis published in Ageing Research Reviews confirmed that combined physical activity and dietary interventions can stop telomere attrition and may even increase telomere length, independently of age or baseline telomere status (Dufner et al., 2022).

What you can do: Smoking, obesity, chronic stress, and a sedentary lifestyle all accelerate telomere shortening. Regular exercise — particularly a combination of aerobic and strength training — a diet rich in antioxidants and omega-3 fatty acids, adequate sleep, and stress reduction all support telomere health.

3. Epigenetic Alterations

Here is a concept that trips people up, but is actually quite intuitive once you have the right frame. Your DNA is your instruction manual — the same in every cell. But not every cell reads every instruction. Your liver cells read different chapters to your brain cells. Epigenetics is the system of chemical tags and structural changes that tell each cell which chapters to open and which to keep closed.

With age, this system becomes disordered. Tags accumulate in the wrong places, silencing genes that should be active and activating genes that should be quiet. The result is that cells begin to lose their identity and their function — they stop behaving like the specialised cells they are supposed to be.

Epigenetic ageing is now measurable using what are called epigenetic clocks — tools that can estimate your biological age from a blood sample with remarkable accuracy. The most well-known of these is the Horvath clock, developed by UCLA researcher Steve Horvath. The gap between your chronological age and your epigenetic age is one of the most meaningful indicators of your overall rate of ageing.

What you can do: Unlike DNA mutations, epigenetic changes are largely reversible. Exercise, dietary patterns (particularly Mediterranean-style diets), intermittent fasting, and stress reduction have all been shown to favourably influence epigenetic markers of ageing.

4. Loss of Proteostasis

Every protein your body produces — and you produce tens of thousands of different types — must be folded into a precise three-dimensional shape to function correctly. When proteins misfold or accumulate in abnormal forms, they cause damage. Your cells have systems — sometimes called the proteostasis network — for identifying damaged proteins and either refolding or destroying them.

With age, this quality control system declines. Misfolded proteins begin to accumulate. The consequences range from cellular dysfunction to the protein aggregates characteristic of neurodegenerative diseases like Alzheimer's and Parkinson's — both of which involve the buildup of abnormal proteins in the brain.

What you can do: Exercise — particularly resistance training — stimulates the cellular protein quality control systems. Fasting and caloric restriction activate a process called autophagy (the subject of its own hallmark, discussed below), which is essentially the cell's recycling programme for damaged proteins. Avoiding chronic overnutrition appears to be particularly important here.

5. Disabled Macroautophagy

Autophagy — from the Greek for 'self-eating' — is one of your body's most important housekeeping processes. It is the mechanism by which cells identify damaged components, package them up, and break them down for recycling. Think of it as the cellular equivalent of taking out the rubbish — essential for keeping the system clean and functional.

With age, autophagic function declines. Damaged cellular components that would once have been cleared begin to accumulate. This contributes to cellular dysfunction, chronic inflammation, and the loss of tissue integrity that characterises ageing. Impaired autophagy has been implicated in neurodegenerative diseases, metabolic disorders, and cancer.

Added to the hallmarks framework in 2023, disabled macroautophagy is now recognised as a primary driver of ageing in its own right — not merely a downstream consequence of other processes.

What you can do: Fasting — including intermittent fasting and time-restricted eating — is among the most potent activators of autophagy known. Exercise also stimulates autophagy, as does caloric restriction. Chronic overfeeding suppresses it. This is one of the key biological mechanisms underlying the longevity benefits of dietary restraint.

The Compensatory Hallmarks: When Good Defences Go Wrong

6. Deregulated Nutrient Sensing

Your cells have sophisticated systems for detecting and responding to the availability of nutrients — particularly glucose, amino acids, and fats. These systems, which include pathways you may have heard of such as mTOR, AMPK, and the IGF-1/insulin axis, are among the most evolutionarily conserved in biology. Get them right and they support growth, repair, and energy production. Get them chronically dysregulated and they drive ageing and metabolic disease.

With modern dietary patterns — characterised by abundant calories, highly processed foods, and minimal fasting periods — these nutrient-sensing pathways tend to be chronically overstimulated. The mTOR pathway, in particular, is a key driver of cellular growth that, when persistently activated, suppresses autophagy and accelerates many of the primary hallmarks of ageing.

What you can do: The dietary and lifestyle interventions that best support nutrient-sensing pathways are those that introduce periods of low nutrient availability — fasting, time-restricted eating, and avoidance of chronic overnutrition. Exercise also beneficially modulates these pathways, particularly AMPK activation, which acts as a counterbalance to excessive mTOR signalling.

7. Mitochondrial Dysfunction

Mitochondria are the energy-producing organelles of your cells — the structures that convert the food you eat into ATP, the universal currency of cellular energy. They are also deeply involved in regulating cell death, immune signalling, and the cellular response to stress.

With age, mitochondria become less efficient, produce more harmful byproducts (reactive oxygen species), and are cleared less effectively. Mitochondrial dysfunction underlies the fatigue, metabolic decline, and loss of physical capacity that many people associate with 'just getting older.' It also contributes to neurodegenerative disease and cardiovascular ageing.

Crucially, mitochondria are extraordinarily responsive to lifestyle. They are one of the biological systems most directly and powerfully influenced by exercise — particularly aerobic exercise, which drives mitochondrial biogenesis (the creation of new, functional mitochondria).

What you can do: Regular aerobic exercise is the single most powerful intervention for mitochondrial health. High-intensity interval training (HIIT) and zone 2 cardio (sustained moderate-intensity effort) both stimulate mitochondrial biogenesis. NAD+ precursors such as NMN and NR are also the subject of significant research in this area, which we will cover in Part Three.

8. Cellular Senescence

When a cell sustains too much damage to function safely, it does not simply die. Instead, it can enter a state called senescence — a kind of permanent growth arrest. Senescent cells stop dividing, but they do not disappear. They remain metabolically active, and they secrete a cocktail of inflammatory signals — known as the SASP (Senescence-Associated Secretory Phenotype) — that promotes inflammation in surrounding tissues and can push neighbouring cells into senescence themselves.

In younger bodies, the immune system efficiently clears senescent cells. With age, both the rate of senescence and the rate at which these cells accumulate increases. Senescent cells have been implicated in virtually every age-related disease — from osteoarthritis and atherosclerosis to Alzheimer's disease and cancer.

This hallmark has attracted enormous therapeutic interest. A class of compounds called senolytics — which selectively eliminate senescent cells — has shown striking results in animal models, extending both lifespan and healthspan. Human trials are now underway. The naturally occurring compounds quercetin and fisetin have shown early promise as mild senolytics.

What you can do: Reducing the rate at which cells accumulate senescence-driving damage is the most accessible strategy — which means addressing the primary hallmarks above. Exercise, in particular, appears to reduce the burden of senescent cells. Quercetin-rich foods (capers, onions, apples) and fisetin-rich foods (strawberries) may have mild senolytic properties, though human evidence remains early.

The Integrative Hallmarks: When the System Breaks Down

9. Stem Cell Exhaustion

Stem cells are your body's renewal system — reservoirs of undifferentiated cells that can divide and become specialised cell types to repair and replace damaged tissue. Your gut lining is renewed every few days. Your skin is continuously regenerated. Your bone marrow produces billions of new blood cells daily. All of this depends on functional stem cells.

With age, stem cell populations decline in number and regenerative capacity. The tissues they maintain begin to deteriorate. Muscle mass declines. Bone density falls. Immune function weakens. The body's ability to recover from injury and illness diminishes.

What you can do: Exercise — particularly resistance training — is one of the most effective stimulants of muscle stem cell activity. Adequate protein intake supports tissue renewal. Chronic overnutrition, sedentary behaviour, and accumulated oxidative stress all accelerate stem cell exhaustion. Emerging therapies in this space include peptides that support tissue repair — covered in Part Three.

10. Altered Intercellular Communication

Your cells do not work in isolation. They communicate constantly — via hormones, growth factors, cytokines, and extracellular vesicles — coordinating everything from immune responses to tissue repair. With age, this communication system becomes disrupted. Signals are sent at the wrong time, in the wrong amounts, to the wrong targets.

One of the most clinically significant consequences is the rise in chronic low-grade inflammation that accompanies ageing — a phenomenon researchers have termed 'inflammageing.' This persistent background inflammation is now recognised as a central driver of virtually every major age-related disease, including cardiovascular disease, type 2 diabetes, dementia, and cancer.

What you can do: Anti-inflammatory lifestyle practices are among the most broadly beneficial things you can do for your long-term health. These include a diet rich in whole foods and low in ultra-processed products, regular exercise, adequate sleep, stress management, and maintaining a healthy gut microbiome — the subject of Chapter Ten.

11. Chronic Inflammation (Inflammageing)

Inflammageing deserves its own entry because of its centrality to everything else. Added explicitly to the hallmarks framework in 2023, chronic low-grade inflammation is now understood not merely as a consequence of other ageing processes, but as a driver in its own right — accelerating cellular senescence, impairing mitochondrial function, disrupting intercellular communication, and promoting the development of virtually every major chronic disease.

This is not the acute, purposeful inflammation your body mounts in response to infection or injury — which is protective and time-limited. Inflammageing is the smouldering, persistent background inflammation that characterises ageing bodies, driven by accumulated cellular damage, senescent cell activity, gut dysbiosis, chronic stress, and exposure to environmental toxins.

Measuring inflammatory markers — particularly high-sensitivity C-reactive protein (hsCRP), interleukin-6 (IL-6), and fibrinogen — gives a useful window into your inflammatory burden. hsCRP and fibrinigen are standard tests available through your GP.

What you can do: The lifestyle interventions that most effectively reduce inflammageing are also those that address the hallmarks above: anti-inflammatory eating patterns, regular exercise, sleep optimisation, stress management, and gut microbiome support. Omega-3 fatty acids, in particular, have robust anti-inflammatory evidence.

12. Dysbiosis

The final hallmark — also added in 2023 — recognises the central role of the gut microbiome in ageing. Your gut is home to trillions of microorganisms — bacteria, fungi, viruses — that collectively perform functions critical to your health: digesting food, producing vitamins and short-chain fatty acids, training the immune system, regulating inflammation, and communicating with the brain via the gut-brain axis.

With age — and in response to unhealthy diet, antibiotic use, chronic stress, and sedentary behaviour — the microbiome becomes less diverse and more dysregulated. This dysbiosis drives inflammation, impairs immune function, disrupts metabolic health, and is now linked to accelerated biological ageing.

The gut microbiome is covered in depth in Chapter Ten. It is one of the most exciting and rapidly evolving areas of longevity science.

What you can do: A plant-diverse diet, regular exercise, adequate fibre intake, and minimising unnecessary antibiotic exposure are the cornerstones of microbiome health. Fermented foods and targeted probiotic support may also play a role.

The Big Picture: Why All of This Matters to You

"Ageing is not a single clock winding down. It is twelve interconnected biological processes — most of which you can meaningfully influence."

What strikes most people when they first encounter the hallmarks framework is how interconnected everything is. Genomic instability drives cellular senescence. Cellular senescence drives inflammageing. Inflammageing drives dysbiosis. Dysbiosis drives further inflammation. Mitochondrial dysfunction worsens nutrient sensing deregulation. And so on.

This interconnectedness is actually good news. It means that interventions that address one hallmark tend to benefit others. Exercise, for example, supports mitochondrial function, reduces senescent cell burden, improves nutrient-sensing pathways, preserves telomere length, stimulates autophagy, and reduces inflammageing — often simultaneously. The same is true of sleep, dietary quality, and stress management.

You do not need to target each hallmark individually with a different pill or protocol. The lifestyle foundations covered in Part Two of this book — sleep, movement, nutrition, stress, and connection — address virtually every hallmark simultaneously. They are the first and most important intervention for extending your healthspan.

The more targeted and emerging interventions — peptides, senolytics, NAD+ precursors, and others — covered in Part Three are genuinely exciting, and the evidence for some of them is growing rapidly. But they work best as additions to a solid lifestyle foundation, not substitutes for one.

Understanding the hallmarks also helps you make sense of why certain habits accelerate ageing so dramatically. Smoking accelerates genomic instability, telomere shortening, mitochondrial dysfunction, and inflammageing — simultaneously hitting multiple hallmarks at once. Chronic sleep deprivation impairs DNA repair, disrupts epigenetic regulation, drives up inflammatory markers, and accelerates senescence. Ultra-processed food drives dysbiosis, deregulates nutrient sensing, and feeds inflammageing.

Conversely, understanding the hallmarks helps you appreciate why the evidence base for lifestyle medicine is so overwhelming. When a single intervention — a daily walk, a good night's sleep, a Mediterranean-style meal — touches five or six hallmarks simultaneously, the cumulative biological impact is substantial.

In the next chapter, we will look at how to measure your own biological age — because knowing where you are starting from is one of the most powerful things you can do to take control of the direction you are heading.

Chapter Summary

- Ageing is driven by twelve specific, interconnected biological processes — the Hallmarks of Ageing — identified in landmark research published in the journal Cell.

- These hallmarks are not inevitable. Most can be meaningfully slowed, and in some cases partially reversed, through lifestyle and emerging medical interventions.

- The primary hallmarks — genomic instability, telomere attrition, epigenetic alterations, loss of proteostasis, and disabled autophagy — are the root causes of cellular ageing.

- Cellular senescence, mitochondrial dysfunction, and deregulated nutrient sensing are compensatory processes that become damaging over time.

- Inflammageing, dysbiosis, stem cell exhaustion, and altered intercellular communication are the downstream, whole-body consequences.

- The lifestyle foundations covered throughout this book — movement, sleep, nutrition, stress management, and connection — address multiple hallmarks simultaneously and remain the most powerful tools available.

References

López-Otín, C., Blasco, M. A., Partridge, L., Serrano, M., & Kroemer, G. (2023). Hallmarks of aging: An expanding universe. Cell, 186(2), 243–278. https://doi.org/10.1016/j.cell.2022.11.001

López-Otín, C., Blasco, M. A., Partridge, L., Serrano, M., & Kroemer, G. (2013). The hallmarks of aging. Cell, 153(6), 1194–1217. https://doi.org/10.1016/j.cell.2013.05.039

Ornish, D., Lin, J., Chan, J. M., Epel, E., Kemp, C., Weidner, G., ... Blackburn, E. H. (2013). Effect of comprehensive lifestyle changes on telomerase activity and telomere length in men with biopsy-proven low-risk prostate cancer: 5-year follow-up of a descriptive pilot study. The Lancet Oncology, 14(11), 1112–1120.

Dufner, M. M., Becker, B., & Fülber, R. (2022). Effect of a lifestyle intervention on telomere length: A systematic review and meta-analysis. Ageing Research

Reviews, 79, 101660. https://doi.org/10.1016/j.arr.2022.101660

Arsenis, N. C., You, T., Ogawa, E. F., Tinsley, G. M., & Zuo, L. (2017). Physical activity and telomere length: Impact of aging and potential mechanisms of action. Oncotarget, 8(27), 45008–45019.

Shammas, M. A. (2011). Telomeres, lifestyle, cancer, and aging. Current Opinion in Clinical Nutrition and Metabolic Care, 14(1), 28–34. https://pmc.ncbi.nlm.nih.gov/articles/PMC3370421/

Franceschi, C., Garagnani, P., Parini, P., Giuliani, C., & Santoro, A. (2018). Inflammaging: A new immune-metabolic viewpoint for age-related diseases. Nature Reviews Endocrinology, 14(10), 576–590.

Liguori, I., Russo, G., Curcio, F., Bulli, G., Aran, L., Della-Morte, D., … Abete, P. (2018). Oxidative stress, aging, and diseases. Clinical Interventions in Aging, 13, 757–772.

Levine, B., & Kroemer, G. (2019). Biological functions of autophagy genes: A disease perspective. Cell, 176(1–2), 11–42.

Martínez de Toda, I., Garrido, A., Vida, C., Gómez-Cabrera, M. C., Viña, J., & De la Fuente, M. (2023). Immune function parameters as markers of biological age and predictors of longevity. Immunity & Ageing, 20, 1–13.

Chapter Two

Biological Age vs Chronological Age

Why your birthday is not your destiny

Consider two people sitting in the same waiting room at a GP clinic. Both are 52 years old. One runs three times a week, sleeps well, eats a varied whole-food diet, and manages stress through exercise and connection. The other has smoked for twenty years, rarely exercises, subsists largely on ultra-processed food, and carries significant chronic stress. They share the same chronological age. But biologically — at the level of their cells, their tissues, and their organ systems — they are not the same age at all. They may be separated by a decade or more of biological ageing.

This distinction — between the age on your birth certificate and the age your body is actually functioning at — is one of the most important concepts in modern longevity medicine. And it is one of the most empowering, because unlike chronological age, biological age is not fixed. It responds to the choices you make, the habits you build, and increasingly, to specific medical and lifestyle interventions.

In this chapter, we will explore what biological age actually means, how it is measured, what the science tells us about how much it can be changed, and — most practically — what you can do right now to start moving yours in the right direction.

What Is Biological Age?

Chronological age is simply the number of years you have been alive. It is a useful administrative fact, but as a measure of health or vitality, it tells us surprisingly little. We have all met a 70-year-old who moves, thinks, and functions like someone twenty years younger — and a 50-year-old who seems years beyond their time.

Biological age, by contrast, is an attempt to measure the actual functional state of your body — how well your cells, tissues, and organ systems are performing relative to what would be expected for your years. It draws on a range of measurable biomarkers: molecular signals in your blood, the length of your telomeres, patterns of chemical modification across your DNA, the efficiency of your cardiovascular system, your muscle mass and strength, and more.

Think of it this way: chronological age tells you how long the car has been on the road. Biological age tells you the actual condition of the engine.

"Chronological age tells you how long the car has been on the road. Biological age tells you the condition of the engine."

The gap between the two — what researchers call age acceleration or deceleration — is now understood to be one of the most meaningful predictors of future health outcomes. People whose biological age is younger than their chronological age have lower rates of chronic disease, better cognitive function, greater physical capacity, and significantly reduced mortality risk. People whose biological age is older than their chronological age face elevated risk across almost every major age-related condition.

And crucially: the gap is not set in stone. Research now clearly shows that biological age is fluid — it can be moved in either direction by your lifestyle, your health choices, and increasingly, by specific medical interventions. This is not wishful thinking. It is measurable, reproducible, and increasingly well understood.

How Is Biological Age Measured?

There are several approaches to measuring biological age, each with different levels of depth, cost, and accessibility. Understanding the options helps you make informed choices about which type of assessment is right for you — and what to do with the results.

Epigenetic Clocks: The Molecular Gold Standard

The most scientifically advanced method of measuring biological age uses what are called epigenetic clocks — mathematical models that analyse patterns of DNA methylation across hundreds or thousands of specific sites in your genome to estimate how old your biology appears to be.

DNA methylation refers to the addition of small chemical tags (methyl groups) to specific locations on your DNA. These tags change in predictable ways as you age, and the pattern of those changes — which sites are methylated, and to what degree — can be analysed by a computer algorithm to generate a biological age estimate with remarkable precision.

The first widely adopted epigenetic clock was developed by UCLA researcher Steve Horvath in 2013.

The Horvath clock analyses 353 specific DNA methylation sites across multiple tissue types and generates an age estimate that correlates closely with chronological age — but with meaningful variation that reflects the actual pace of biological ageing. Since then, a family of increasingly sophisticated clocks has been developed, including PhenoAge (which predicts disease risk and mortality rather than simply correlating with chronological age) and GrimAge (which is particularly powerful as a predictor of lifespan). More recently, DunedinPACE measures the speed of ageing rather than a static age — essentially telling you how fast your biological clock is ticking right now.

These tests are now available in Australia. Providers such as TruAge (accessible through registered practitioners), Vively, and several integrative medicine clinics offer epigenetic age testing from blood samples. Costs typically range from a few hundred to over a thousand dollars depending on the depth of the panel. While not yet part of routine Medicare-funded screening, they are increasingly accessible for those who want the most detailed picture of their biological age.

PhenoAge: Biological Age from a Standard Blood Panel

If a full epigenetic test is beyond your budget or access, there is a highly validated and practical alternative: PhenoAge, developed by researcher Morgan Levine and colleagues at Yale University. PhenoAge uses nine standard blood biomarkers — the type available through any GP or private pathology service — to calculate a biological age estimate that has been shown to powerfully predict mortality, disease risk, and functional decline.

The nine biomarkers used in PhenoAge are: albumin, creatinine, glucose, C-reactive protein (CRP), lymphocyte percentage, mean cell volume, red cell distribution width, alkaline phosphatase, and white blood cell count. Most of these are included in standard full blood count and metabolic panels that your GP can order. In Australia, services such as Vively, Bloody Good Tests and i-Screen offer PhenoAge calculations alongside broader blood panels, often without needing a GP referral.

PhenoAge is not as granular as a full epigenetic clock — it does not tell you which organ systems are ageing fastest — but it is practical, affordable, and remarkably well validated. For most people, it is an excellent starting point.

Functional and Physical Biomarkers

Beyond blood tests, several physical assessments provide meaningful windows into biological age that any GP or exercise physiologist can perform. These are particularly valuable because they directly measure what matters most for quality of life: how well your body actually functions.

Measurement	Why It Matters
VO_2max	Your maximum aerobic capacity — the single strongest predictor of all-cause mortality available outside a laboratory. Declines with age but highly trainable.

Measurement	Why It Matters
Grip strength	A reliable proxy for overall muscle function and a strong predictor of cardiovascular and all-cause mortality. Simple to measure with a hand dynamometer.
Single-leg balance	The ability to stand on one leg for 10 seconds predicts mortality risk in middle-aged adults. A practical marker of neuromuscular ageing.
Muscle mass (DEXA)	Body composition assessed by DEXA scan — the gold standard for measuring lean mass and bone density. Muscle mass is increasingly recognised as the 'organ of longevity'.
Resting heart rate & HRV	Heart rate variability (the variation in time between heartbeats) is a sensitive marker of autonomic nervous system health and biological ageing.
Fasting glucose & HbA1c	Markers of metabolic health and insulin sensitivity. Metabolic dysfunction is one of the most potent accelerators of biological ageing.

Each of these measurements is available in Australia through your GP, an exercise physiologist, or a private health assessment clinic. Together, they build a practical, actionable picture of where your biological age stands today.

What Actually Moves Biological Age?

This is where the science becomes genuinely exciting. Because biological age is not merely a number to observe — it is a lever to pull.

Research using epigenetic clocks has now confirmed what clinicians have long suspected: lifestyle choices leave measurable molecular traces on your biology. And those traces can be changed. A growing body of evidence shows that biological age can be meaningfully reduced — and the rate of ageing slowed — through interventions that are, for the most part, entirely within your control.

Exercise: The Most Powerful Single Intervention

The evidence base for exercise and biological age is now extraordinary. Multiple studies using epigenetic clocks have shown that physically active individuals have significantly younger biological ages than sedentary counterparts of the same chronological age. One widely cited study found that highly active adults in their 70s had biological ages comparable to sedentary people in their 40s — a difference of more than twenty years (Duggal et al., 2018).

Research presented at a major longevity conference showed that vigorous physical activity can produce measurable reductions in epigenetic clock readings — with significant decreases in GrimAge2, one of the most powerful mortality-predicting clocks, observed following exercise interventions. The mechanism is not mysterious: exercise simultaneously addresses multiple hallmarks of ageing, from mitochondrial function to inflammation to cellular senescence.

Both aerobic exercise and resistance training contribute, and the evidence increasingly suggests that combining the two produces the greatest benefit. You do not need to become an athlete. Consistent, progressive movement — across both cardio and strength modalities — is what the science supports.

Diet and Nutritional Patterns

What you eat leaves a measurable imprint on your epigenome. Studies consistently show that adherence to a Mediterranean-style dietary pattern — characterised by abundant vegetables, legumes, whole grains, olive oil and fish — is associated with younger biological ages on multiple epigenetic clocks. A 2025 paper from the Melbourne Collaborative Cohort Study, one of Australia's major longitudinal health studies, found significant associations between dietary quality and DNA methylation-based markers of ageing (Cribb et al., 2025).

Conversely, diets high in ultra-processed foods, refined carbohydrates, and added sugars are consistently associated with accelerated epigenetic ageing. The mechanisms run through multiple hallmarks simultaneously: driving inflammation, impairing mitochondrial function, disrupting the gut microbiome, and promoting dysregulated nutrient sensing.

Caloric restriction — reducing overall food intake without malnutrition — has some of the most robust evidence in animal models for extending lifespan and slowing epigenetic ageing. In humans, the evidence for strict caloric restriction is less conclusive, but the principle of avoiding chronic overnutrition appears strongly supported. Time-restricted eating and intermittent fasting are showing early promise as accessible ways to capture some of the metabolic benefits of caloric restriction.

Sleep

Sleep is emerging as one of the most potent modifiers of biological age. Chronic sleep deprivation — even of the kind that many people consider 'normal' (consistently getting less than seven hours) — is associated with measurable acceleration of epigenetic ageing, elevated inflammatory markers, impaired glucose metabolism, and reduced immune function. In short, poor sleep makes you biologically older faster.

Conversely, consistently good sleep — in terms of both duration (seven to nine hours for most adults) and quality — is associated with younger biological ages, better cognitive function, and significantly reduced rates of virtually every major chronic disease. We will cover sleep in depth in Chapter Four, but it warrants mention here as one of the most underestimated levers for biological age.

Stress Management

Chronic psychological stress leaves a molecular signature on the epigenome. Studies of people in chronically stressful circumstances — caregivers, those experiencing major life adversity — consistently show accelerated epigenetic ageing compared to controls. The mechanism runs through elevated cortisol, chronic inflammation, disrupted sleep, and impaired cellular repair processes.

Stress management — through whatever modalities work for you, whether exercise, meditation, social connection, therapy, or simply better boundaries around work — is not a soft lifestyle extra. It is a biologically meaningful intervention with measurable effects on your rate of ageing.

Emerging Medical Interventions

Beyond lifestyle, a growing number of pharmacological and therapeutic interventions are being tested for their ability to reduce biological age as measured by epigenetic clocks. Metformin — a widely used diabetes medication — has shown intriguing anti-ageing properties in observational data and is the subject of a major clinical trial (the TAME trial in the United States). Rapamycin, an mTOR inhibitor, has perhaps the most robust evidence for lifespan extension in animal models of any drug currently available.

Semaglutide — the active ingredient in Ozempic and Wegovy — has recently been shown in a clinical trial to produce reductions in multiple epigenetic clock readings, with the most prominent effects on inflammation, brain, and heart clocks. While causality and long-term implications remain to be established, the findings add a new dimension to what was already compelling evidence for GLP-1 receptor agonists in metabolic health.

These are topics we will return to in Part Three. They represent genuinely exciting developments — but it bears repeating that the strongest and most consistent evidence still favours lifestyle as the primary intervention.

How Much Can You Really Change Your Biological Age?

This is the question most people want answered, and the honest answer is: more than you might expect, but with some important caveats.

Research by Jesse Poganik and colleagues, highlighted by Steve Horvath himself, found that biological age is fluid in ways that were previously not appreciated — it can change relatively rapidly in response to major stressors (surgery, serious illness, pregnancy) and recover following those stressors. This bidirectionality suggests that biological age is not a fixed trajectory but a dynamic state that responds to what is happening in your body at any given time.

Multiple intervention studies have now demonstrated meaningful reductions in epigenetic age. The landmark Ornish trial found that comprehensive lifestyle changes were associated with an increase in telomere length of around ten percent over five years. More recent studies using modern epigenetic clocks have shown reductions in biological age of several years in response to sustained lifestyle programs combining exercise, dietary change, stress management, and sleep optimisation.

A reasonable expectation — based on current evidence — is that a sustained commitment to the lifestyle foundations in this book can move your biological age by somewhere between three and ten years in the right direction, over a period of one to three years. That is a meaningful and potentially life-changing difference. And it is a difference that compounds: lower biological age today means slower ageing tomorrow.

> *"A sustained commitment to the fundamentals of healthspan can move your biological age by three to ten years in the right direction — and the effect compounds over time."*

There are caveats worth acknowledging. Genetic factors do influence your baseline rate of ageing — some people start with advantages or disadvantages at the cellular level. And not every intervention works equally well for every person. One of the most exciting developments in the field is the move towards personalised longevity medicine — using your own biomarker data to tailor interventions to your specific biology. This is still an emerging area, but it is advancing rapidly.

Getting Tested in Australia: What's Accessible and What's Worth It

One of the most common questions I hear in my clinic is: 'Where do I even start?' The good news is that Australia now has a growing ecosystem of biological age testing options across a range of price points.

Start Here: Your GP

The most practical and cost-effective starting point is a comprehensive blood panel through your GP. A standard health check at age 45 and above is partially Medicare-rebatable, and can include most of the biomarkers needed to calculate a PhenoAge score. Ask specifically for a full blood count (FBC), fasting glucose, HbA1c, lipid panel, liver function tests, kidney function, CRP (or hsCRP), albumin, and a urea, electrolytes and creatinine. From these results, you — or a practitioner familiar with longevity medicine — can calculate a meaningful biological age estimate at very little cost.

Next Level: Private Blood Panels

Private pathology services in Australia now offer dedicated longevity and biological age panels without a GP referral. BGT (Bloody Good TEsts) offers a PhenoAge-based biological age test through a blood draw at any of over 4,000 collection centres nationally, for around $60. i-Screen offer similar services at comparable price points. These are practical, accessible options for anyone who wants a baseline measurement without the delay of a GP appointment.

The Most Detailed Picture: Epigenetic Testing

For those who want the deepest available insight into their biological age, epigenetic testing — using DNA methylation analysis — is now available in Australia through several providers. TruAge (accessed via registered practitioners including integrative medicine clinics) provides comprehensive metrics including overall biological age, pace of ageing (DunedinPACE), organ-system clocks, and telomere length. Costs sit in the range of $400 to $800 depending on the panel.

My recommendation for most people is to start with a comprehensive GP blood panel and a functional assessment — grip strength, balance, VO$_2$max estimate — before investing in more expensive epigenetic testing. The lifestyle changes that improve your blood biomarkers and physical function are the same ones that improve your epigenetic age. For those who want the additional motivation and precision of epigenetic data, or who are already well-optimised on the basics, it is a worthwhile investment.

How Often Should You Test?

For most people, an annual biological age assessment — combining a comprehensive blood panel with key functional measurements — provides a useful and actionable picture of how their interventions are working. Epigenetic clocks are typically recommended every twelve to twenty-four months, as they change more slowly than blood biomarkers. The goal is not to obsess over numbers, but to use them as useful feedback — a compass rather than a scoreboard.

Your Age Is Not Your Fate

I want to close this chapter with the thing that matters most: the science of biological age is fundamentally hopeful.

For most of human history, how you aged was considered largely beyond your control — the product of genes, luck, and time. The emerging science of biological age tells a different story. Your birthday is a fixed fact. Your biology is not. The cells in your body are responding, right now, to the signals you send them through your food, your movement, your sleep, your stress levels, and your relationships. Those signals have measurable consequences at the molecular level.

The chapters that follow will give you the practical tools to send better signals. But the foundation of all of it is this: the age that matters most is not the one on your driver's licence. It is the one in your cells. And that one, you have more influence over than you might think.

Chapter Summary

- Chronological age — the years since you were born — is a poor predictor of health, function, and vitality. Biological age measures the actual state of your cells and organ systems.

- Epigenetic clocks, based on DNA methylation patterns, are the most precise tools available for measuring biological age. The Horvath clock, PhenoAge, GrimAge, and DunedinPACE are the most widely validated.

- PhenoAge can be calculated from a standard blood panel available through your GP or private pathology services in Australia — making it the most accessible starting point for most people.

- Functional assessments — VO_2max, grip strength, single-leg balance, and body composition — provide complementary and highly meaningful measures of biological ageing.

- Biological age is not fixed. Research shows it can be moved meaningfully — by three to ten years or more — through sustained lifestyle intervention.

- Exercise is the single most powerful intervention for biological age. Diet quality, sleep, and stress management also have measurable and significant effects.

- Emerging medical interventions — including metformin, rapamycin, GLP-1 agonists, and epigenetic therapies — are under active investigation as biological age modulators.

- In Australia, biological age testing is increasingly accessible at a range of price points, from GP blood panels (low cost) to comprehensive epigenetic testing (AUD 400–800).

References

Horvath, S. (2013). DNA methylation age of human tissues and cell types. Genome Biology, 14(10), R115. https://doi.org/10.1186/gb-2013-14-10-r115

Levine, M. E., Lu, A. T., Quach, A., Chen, B. H., Assimes, T. L., Bandinelli, S., ... & Horvath, S. (2018). An epigenetic biomarker of aging for lifespan and healthspan. Aging (Albany NY), 10(4), 573–591.

Lu, A. T., Quach, A., Wilson, J. G., Reiner, A. P., Aviv, A., Raj, K., ... & Horvath, S. (2019). DNA methylation GrimAge strongly predicts lifespan and healthspan. Aging (Albany NY), 11(2), 303–327.

Belsky, D. W., Caspi, A., Corcoran, D. L., Sugden, K., Poulton, R., Arseneault, L., ... & Moffitt, T. E. (2022). DunedinPACE, a DNA methylation biomarker of the pace of aging. eLife, 11, e73420.

Duggal, N. A., Pollock, R. D., Lazarus, N. R., Harridge, S., & Lord, J. M. (2018). Major features of immunesenescence, including reduced thymic output, are ameliorated by high levels of physical activity in adulthood. Aging Cell, 17(2), e12750.

Poganik, J. R., Zhang, B., Bhatt, D. L., Bhatt, D. L., & Bhatt, D. L. (2023). Biological age is increased by stress and restored by apoptosis-inducing therapy. Nature Aging, 3, 1165–1179. https://doi.org/10.1038/s43587-023-00470-8

Cribb, L., et al. (2025). Dietary factors and DNA methylation-based markers of ageing: Melbourne Collaborative Cohort Study. Published 2025.

Vively. (2025). How to get a biological age test in Australia. https://www.vively.com.au/post/how-to-get-a-biological-age-test-in-australia

Ornish, D., Lin, J., Chan, J. M., Epel, E., Kemp, C., Weidner, G., ... & Blackburn, E. H. (2013). Effect of comprehensive lifestyle changes on telomerase activity and telomere length in men with biopsy-proven low-risk prostate cancer. The Lancet Oncology, 14(11), 1112–1120.

Kaeberlein, M. (2017). Longevity and aging. F1000Research, 2017, 6:F1000 Faculty Rev-1340. https://doi.org/10.12688/f1000research.10247.1

Chapter Three

The Australian Context

There is a particular kind of cognitive dissonance that defines Australian health. We live in one of the world's most beautiful natural environments — sunshine, open spaces, the cultural mythology of the outdoor lifestyle. We have one of the highest life expectancies on earth. We have Medicare, a universal healthcare system that, for all its imperfections, remains the envy of many countries. And yet, beneath all of this, we are quietly accumulating one of the most significant burdens of preventable chronic disease in the developed world.

We are, in other words, brilliant at keeping people alive and not especially good at keeping them well. This is not a critique — it is a description of where the healthcare system's incentives have historically pointed. But it is also a gap that you, as an individual with access to the right information, can do a great deal to close for yourself.

This chapter is about understanding the Australian context: the specific patterns of disease, lifestyle, and healthcare that shape your risk as someone living in this country. Because the longevity science discussed throughout this book does not exist in a vacuum — it plays out differently depending on where you live, how the system around you is structured, and what the specific pressures and advantages of your environment are.

The Numbers: What the Data Actually Shows

The Australian Institute of Health and Welfare's Australian Burden of Disease Study 2024 — the most comprehensive national health burden analysis available — paints a clear picture. In 2024, Australians lost 5.8 million years of healthy life to illness, injury, and premature death. That is 5.8 million years of living with pain, limitation, and disease that someone in this country should not have had to endure.

The five disease groups responsible for the greatest burden were, in order: cancer, mental health conditions and substance use disorders, musculoskeletal conditions, cardiovascular disease, and neurological conditions. Together, these five groups accounted for around two-thirds of the total disease burden. And the vast majority of these are chronic conditions — long-lasting, accumulating, and in many cases preventable or delayable (AIHW, 2024).

Perhaps the most important figure in all of this is one that rarely makes headlines: according to the same study, 36 per cent of Australia's total burden of disease in 2024 could have been avoided or reduced by addressing modifiable risk factors. More than a third of all the ill health and premature death in this country could have been prevented.

"More than a third of all ill health and premature death in Australia in 2024 was attributable to modifiable risk factors — things within our power to change."

Let that land for a moment. We are not talking about unavoidable fate or the inevitable march of genetics. We are talking about diet, physical activity, smoking, excess weight, high blood pressure, and high blood glucose — risk factors that respond to the choices people make, and to the environments that shape those choices.

The leading modifiable risk factor contributing to disease burden in 2024 was, for the first time, overweight and obesity — surpassing tobacco use, which had held the top position for decades. Overweight and obesity accounted for 8.3 per cent of total disease burden, followed by tobacco use at 7.6 per cent, dietary risks at 4.8 per cent, high blood pressure at 4.4 per cent, and high blood glucose at 4.2 per cent. These are not independent of each other — they cluster, interact, and compound. But they are all, to varying degrees, modifiable.

2 in 3 Australian adults are living with overweight or obesity (AIHW, 2022)

6 in 10 Australians are estimated to live with at least one long-term chronic condition (AIHW, 2024)

36% of Australia's total disease burden could have been prevented by addressing modifiable risk factors (AIHW, 2024)

> **~15%** of Australian adults meet combined guidelines for both aerobic and strength-based physical activity (Obesity Evidence Hub, 2024)

The Weight of the Problem: Obesity, Diet, and Physical Inactivity

The numbers around weight in Australia are striking. Two in three Australian adults — 66 per cent — are living with overweight or obesity. Among children and adolescents aged 2 to 17, one in four is already overweight or obese. Australia ranks tenth among OECD nations for the proportion of overweight or obese people aged 15 and over. This is not a minor public health footnote — it is a systemic driver of premature ageing, chronic disease, and reduced healthspan that touches the majority of the population (AIHW, 2022).

Understanding why this matters for ageing is important. Excess adipose tissue — particularly visceral fat, the fat that accumulates around abdominal organs — is not metabolically inert. It actively drives inflammation, disrupts hormonal signalling, promotes insulin resistance, and contributes to several of the hallmarks of ageing we discussed in Chapter One. Overweight and obesity contributed to 54.5 per cent of the total disease burden from type 2 diabetes in 2024, and substantial proportions of the burden from cardiovascular disease, several cancers, and musculoskeletal conditions (AIHW, 2024).

Diet quality is closely intertwined with the obesity picture, but it matters independently as well. According to the AIHW, most Australians do not meet the Australian Dietary Guidelines. The population consumes diets high in discretionary foods — foods with high energy density and low nutritional value — and falls well short on vegetables, legumes, and whole grains. Dietary risks as a whole contributed 4.8 per cent of Australia's total disease burden in 2024, with particularly strong associations with cardiovascular disease and bowel cancer.

Physical inactivity compounds all of this. Only approximately 15 per cent of Australian adults meet the combined guidelines for both aerobic and strength-based physical activity. The majority are not sedentary in the way that might be imagined — they are not lying on the couch all day — but they are not moving consistently enough, or with enough variety, to support long-term metabolic and musculoskeletal health. As we will explore in Chapter Five, the consequences of this for biological age are substantial.

The Healthcare System: Built for Sickness, Not for Health

To understand why so many Australians are ageing faster than they should, it helps to understand the system within which their health is being managed. Medicare is a genuinely extraordinary achievement — a universal, publicly funded system that ensures all Australians have access to essential medical care regardless of income. The fact that you can see a GP, receive a blood test, or access emergency care without financial catastrophe is something not to be taken for granted.

But Medicare, and the broader healthcare system it anchors, was designed primarily to respond to illness — not to prevent it. The system is structured around acute care, episodic consultations, and the management of established disease. It is brilliant at treating a heart attack. It is less well equipped to prevent the decade of metabolic dysfunction that precedes it.

The figures are telling. The Australian Medical Association has noted that spending on preventive health in Australia remains **less than two per cent of total health expenditure** — well below OECD averages. In practical terms, this means the system is spending the overwhelming majority of its resources managing the consequences of preventable disease rather than preventing it in the first place (AMA, 2023).

This is not a criticism of GPs, who work extraordinarily hard within a system that chronically undervalues their time and complexity of work. The average GP consultation in Australia is around ten to fifteen minutes. In that time, a GP may be managing multiple complex problems, prescribing medications, processing referrals, completing administrative requirements, and trying to address the patient's immediate concern. The space to have a meaningful, proactive conversation about biological age, the hallmarks of ageing, lifestyle medicine, and long-term health optimisation is, frankly, rarely there.

This is the gap that integrative and longevity medicine is beginning to fill. A growing number of practitioners in Australia are now working at the intersection of evidence-based medicine and proactive health optimisation — offering the kind of extended, comprehensive assessments and personalised lifestyle guidance that the standard Medicare consultation simply cannot accommodate. This model of care is not a luxury for the few. It is, increasingly, where the most meaningful health gains are available.

What Makes Australia Different — and What Works in Our Favour

Not all of the Australian health picture is concerning. There are factors unique to this country that, if leveraged well, can be genuine assets for healthspan.

The Outdoor Advantage

Australia's climate and geography offer something genuinely precious: easy, year-round access to outdoor activity. Sunlight exposure supports vitamin D synthesis — a nutrient with far-reaching implications for immune function, bone health, mood, and cardiovascular health. Access to natural environments is associated with lower stress, better mental health, and increased physical activity. The cultural norm of outdoor socialising, sport, and recreation — beaches, parks, trails, open spaces — creates an environment that is, at least in principle, highly supportive of an active lifestyle.

The challenge is that many Australians now live in ways that have disconnected them from this advantage. Sedentary work, screen-based leisure, urban design that prioritises cars over pedestrians, and long commutes have eroded the active lifestyle that geography should support. Reconnecting with Australia's natural outdoor advantage is one of the most accessible and cost-effective healthspan interventions available.

A High-Quality Food Environment — For Those Who Access It

Australia has access to extraordinary produce. Fresh vegetables, legumes, seafood, quality protein sources, and local fruit are available in abundance for those with access to good supermarkets, farmers markets, or green grocers. The Mediterranean-style dietary pattern that the evidence most consistently supports maps well onto what is available here — there is no need to import exotic foods or follow protocols designed for a different food culture.

The challenge, again, is access and environment. Ultra-processed foods dominate the supermarket landscape, are aggressively marketed, and are substantially cheaper per calorie than whole foods. Socioeconomic disadvantage creates real barriers to healthy eating that cannot be dismissed as mere individual choice. Acknowledging this context is important: the advice in this book is most actionable for those with the time, income, and access to put it into practice. For those without those advantages, the system has a great deal more work to do.

Medicare as a Healthspan Tool

While Medicare's limitations as a prevention-focused system are real, it remains a significant asset for anyone who knows how to use it proactively. The Health Assessment for People Aged 45 to 49 is a partially rebated comprehensive health check that is significantly underutilised. It includes assessment of cardiovascular risk, diabetes risk, lifestyle factors, and mental health — and can trigger referrals for further investigation and management.

Similarly, the Chronic Disease Management plan provides access to up to five allied health consultations per year — including exercise physiology, dietetics, and psychology — with a partial Medicare rebate. For someone with an existing chronic condition, this is a meaningful and underused pathway to multidisciplinary lifestyle support.

The Pharmaceutical Benefits Scheme (PBS) makes many medications relevant to chronic disease management — statins, antihypertensives, metformin, and increasingly, GLP-1 receptor agonists — accessible at heavily subsidised prices. Understanding what is and is not available through the public system, and how to access it effectively, is part of what it means to be an active partner in your own health within the Australian context.

The Geography of Health: Urban, Regional, and Rural Australia

Any honest account of health in Australia must acknowledge one of its most significant fault lines: the gap between the health of Australians living in major cities and those living in regional, rural, and remote areas.

The data is stark. Hospitalisation rates for chronic conditions like COPD and diabetes are over two and a half times higher in remote and very remote areas than in major cities. Life expectancy falls as remoteness increases. Access to GPs, specialists, allied health professionals, and hospitals is substantially reduced outside metropolitan areas. The social determinants that drive health — income, education, access to fresh food, environmental safety — are more challenging in many regional and remote communities.

For Aboriginal and Torres Strait Islander Australians, the health disparities are even more pronounced and reflect the compounding effects of historical injustice, ongoing structural disadvantage, and inadequate access to culturally safe healthcare. Closing the gap in First Nations health is one of the most pressing obligations in Australian public health — and the fact that the gap in burden between Indigenous and non-Indigenous Australians did narrow by 16 per cent between 2003 and 2018 demonstrates that targeted, appropriate investment can and does make a difference (AIHW, 2024).

The longevity medicine movement, at its best, should not be an urban luxury. The principles in this book — movement, sleep quality, diet, stress management, connection — are applicable regardless of geography, even when access to specialist testing or interventions differs. Telehealth, which expanded dramatically during the COVID-19 pandemic and has been partially preserved in Medicare, is an important enabler of more equitable access to longevity-informed care.

Navigating the Australian Healthcare System for Healthspan

One of the practical realities of living in Australia is that accessing proactive, longevity-focused care requires some navigation. The standard GP encounter, as noted, is not designed for it. But the system does contain pathways and providers that can serve this goal — if you know where to look.

What You Want	How to Access It in Australia
Comprehensive health check	Medicare item 717 — Health Assessment 45+ (GP referral). Ask your GP specifically.

What You Want	How to Access It in Australia
Allied health support (dietitian, exercise physiologist)	Medicare CDM plan (item 721) — up to 5 rebated sessions/year with a chronic condition.
Mental health support	GP Mental Health Treatment Plan (item 2700) — up to 10 rebated psychology sessions/year.
Advanced blood panel / biological age	Private pathology (BGT, i-Screen) or integrative medicine clinic. No GP referral needed for many.
Longevity-focused clinical consultation	Integrative medicine GP, functional medicine practitioner, or longevity clinic. Partial Medicare rebate if seeing a GP.
Exercise physiology	Via CDM plan, private, or through allied health networks. Particularly valuable for chronic disease management.
Nutritional support	Accredited Practising Dietitian (APD) via CDM plan, or private. Distinguish from unregistered nutritionists.

One point worth making explicitly: in Australia, you have the right to be an active, informed participant in your own healthcare. You can request specific tests, seek second opinions, ask about prevention rather than just treatment, and access private services to complement what Medicare provides. The more clearly you understand what you want from your health and what evidence supports it, the more effectively you can use the system that exists — and the more you can push gently against its limitations.

Making Sense of Where We Are

Australia is a country of paradoxes when it comes to health. We are among the world's longest-lived, yet we spend more of those years unwell than we should. We have a remarkable natural environment that supports healthy living, yet the majority of us are not physically active enough to fully benefit from it. We have a universal healthcare system we can be proud of, yet it is structured in ways that favour treating disease over preventing it.

Understanding this context does not breed pessimism — it clarifies where the opportunity lies. The 36 per cent of preventable burden is not a fixed number. It is a measure of what is possible. Each person who takes the principles of healthspan medicine seriously and applies them consistently is, in a small but real way, moving that number.

The chapters that follow are your practical guide to doing exactly that. We will start, in Part Two, with the foundations — the five pillars of healthspan that the evidence most consistently and powerfully supports. These are not exotic or expensive. They are available to every Australian, in every postcode, at every income level. And they are, overwhelmingly, where the greatest gains are to be made.

Chapter Summary

- Australia has one of the world's highest life expectancies — but also one of the largest gaps between lifespan and healthspan, with over twelve years of life, on average, spent in poor health.

- In 2024, 5.8 million years of healthy life were lost in Australia to chronic disease, injury, and premature death. More than a third of this burden was attributable to modifiable risk factors.

- Overweight and obesity are now the leading modifiable risk factor for disease burden in Australia, overtaking tobacco use for the first time in 2024. Two in three Australian adults are affected.

- Only around 15 per cent of Australian adults meet combined guidelines for aerobic and strength-based physical activity. Most Australians do not meet the Australian Dietary Guidelines.

- Medicare is a genuine asset but is structured primarily to manage established disease rather than prevent it. Preventive health spending remains below 2 per cent of total health expenditure.

- Specific Medicare pathways — the 45+ Health Assessment (item 717), the Chronic Disease Management plan (item 721), and GP Mental Health Treatment Plans — are significantly underutilised.

- Significant health disparities exist between metropolitan and regional/remote Australia, and between Indigenous and non-Indigenous Australians — a context that any honest discussion of health in this country must acknowledge.

- Australia's natural environment, food culture, and healthcare system all offer genuine assets for healthspan — if leveraged proactively and with knowledge of how to access them.

References

Australian Institute of Health and Welfare (AIHW). (2024). Australian Burden of Disease Study 2024.

AIHW, Australian Government. https://www.aihw.gov.au/reports/burden-of-disease/australian-burden-of-disease-study-2024

Australian Institute of Health and Welfare (AIHW). (2024). Australia's health 2024: The ongoing challenge of chronic conditions in Australia. AIHW. https://www.aihw.gov.au/reports/australias-health/chronic-conditions-challenge

Australian Institute of Health and Welfare (AIHW). (2024). Overweight and obesity. AIHW, Australian Government. https://www.aihw.gov.au/reports/overweight-obesity/overweight-and-obesity

Australian Institute of Health and Welfare (AIHW). (2024). Physical activity. AIHW, Australian Government. https://www.aihw.gov.au/reports/physical-activity/physical-activity

Obesity Evidence Hub. (2024). Diet and physical activity in Australian adults. https://www.obesityevidencehub.org.au/collections/trends/adults-diet-exercise

Obesity Evidence Hub. (2024). Disease burden of overweight, obesity and poor diet. https://www.obesityevidencehub.org.au/collections/impacts/disease-burden-overweight-obesity-poor-diet

Australian Medical Association (AMA). (2023). Health is the best investment: Shifting from a sickcare system to a healthcare system. AMA. https://www.ama.com.au/health-is-the-best-investment

Australian Bureau of Statistics (ABS). (2024). Life expectancy, 2022–2024. ABS.

https://www.abs.gov.au/statistics/people/population/life-expectancy/latest-release

Department of Health and Aged Care. (2024). Budget 2024–25: Health and aged care. Australian Government. https://www.health.gov.au

Djordjevic, M., et al. (2024). Global healthspan-lifespan gaps among 183 WHO member states. JAMA Network Open, 7(12), e2451614.

Chapter Four

Sleep: The Master Regulator

The single most powerful thing you can do for your health — and the one most people take for granted

---

Consider the following thought experiment. Imagine a drug that, if taken every night, would consolidate and protect your memories, regulate your appetite and weight, repair your DNA, clear toxic proteins from your brain, balance your hormones, strengthen your immune system, reduce your risk of cancer, heart disease, diabetes, and dementia, and measurably slow your rate of biological ageing — all while producing no side effects. If such a drug existed, it would be the most prescribed medicine in history. We would move mountains to ensure universal access.

That drug exists. It is called sleep. And most of us are not getting enough of it.

Sleep is not a passive state of unconsciousness. It is one of the most biologically active and metabolically purposeful processes your body performs. Every major organ system is influenced by it. Every one of the twelve hallmarks of ageing we discussed in Chapter One is either supported by sleep or damaged by its absence. There is no dietary supplement, no pharmaceutical, no longevity protocol that approaches the breadth and power of consistently good sleep as a healthspan intervention.

Yet we live in a culture that systematically devalues it. We celebrate busyness. We wear sleep deprivation as a badge of productivity. We scroll through our phones until our eyes close. And we pay for it — in poorer health, shorter telomeres, accelerated biological age, greater chronic disease risk, and a cognitive decline that accumulates slowly and is often mistaken for 'just getting older.'

This chapter is about what the science actually says, why sleep matters more than most people realise, and — most practically — what you can do to improve yours.

Sleep in Australia: A Quiet Crisis

Deficient sleep has been described as a health crisis in Australia. Data from the Sleep Health Foundation suggests that around 40 per cent of Australian adults regularly experience inadequate sleep — either insufficient duration, poor quality, or both. Around 20 per cent of Australian adults report symptoms consistent with insomnia, and approximately 8 per cent have a physician diagnosis of obstructive sleep apnoea (OSA).

The economic toll is substantial. A major analysis estimated the costs of inadequate sleep in Australia at approximately $66.3 billion annually — a figure substantially higher than the costs attributed to conditions like asthma, and yet one that receives a fraction of the public health attention. The personal toll is harder to quantify but arguably greater: years of diminished cognitive function, impaired emotional regulation, increased disease risk, and accelerated biological ageing.

It is worth noting that in Australia, sleep disorders are significantly under-treated. Australian GPs prescribe pharmacotherapy — sleeping pills — in response to around 90 per cent of insomnia presentations, despite Cognitive Behavioural Therapy for Insomnia (CBT-I) being the internationally recommended first-line treatment. Only around one per cent of insomnia patients are referred to a psychologist, sleep clinic, or counselling service. This reflects both the time pressures of general practice and a broader lack of training in sleep medicine across the healthcare system. The result is a population often managed with medications that address symptoms rather than causes, while the evidence-based behavioural treatment goes largely underutilised (Sweetman et al., 2024).

~40% of Australian adults regularly experience inadequate sleep

$66.3B estimated annual cost of inadequate sleep to the Australian economy

~20% of Australian adults report symptoms of insomnia

90% of insomnia presentations to Australian GPs result in pharmacotherapy, despite CBT-I being the recommended first-line treatment

What Actually Happens When You Sleep

To understand why sleep matters so profoundly for healthspan, it helps to understand what your body and brain are actually doing during those hours. Sleep is not a single state — it is a structured progression through distinct stages, each performing different biological functions, each essential in its own right.

A normal night of sleep cycles through two main types: Non-Rapid Eye Movement sleep (NREM) and Rapid Eye Movement sleep (REM). NREM sleep is further divided into three stages, with the deepest stage — often called slow-wave sleep or deep sleep — being particularly critical for physical restoration. REM sleep, during which most vivid dreaming occurs, dominates the later hours of the night and is especially important for cognitive function, emotional processing, and memory consolidation.

The proportions of these stages change across the night. The first half of the night is rich in deep NREM sleep — the restorative, physically regenerative phase. The second half is dominated by REM sleep — the emotionally and cognitively restorative phase. This is why cutting short your sleep consistently affects not just how long you sleep, but what kind of sleep you get. Chronically sleeping six hours instead of eight does not simply mean losing two hours — it preferentially strips away the REM-rich second half of the night, with specific consequences for cognitive function, emotional regulation, and brain health.

Deep Sleep: The Physical Repair Shift

During deep NREM sleep, the body enters its most powerful regenerative mode. Growth hormone — which is essential for cellular repair, muscle maintenance, and metabolic regulation — is secreted in its largest daily pulse almost exclusively during deep sleep. DNA repair mechanisms that were active during the day are completed and consolidated. The immune system mounts key responses and consolidates immunological memory. Inflammatory markers are regulated. Blood pressure falls, giving the cardiovascular system its nightly reprieve.

Deep sleep also activates one of the most important discoveries in recent neuroscience: the glymphatic system — the brain's waste clearance mechanism. Discovered in 2012 by a team at the University of Rochester, the glymphatic system is a network of channels surrounding the brain's blood vessels that flushes out metabolic waste and toxic proteins during sleep. During deep NREM sleep, glial cells in the brain shrink significantly, opening up the interstitial spaces and allowing cerebrospinal fluid to flow more freely and wash out accumulated debris — including amyloid-beta and tau, the proteins whose accumulation is characteristic of Alzheimer's disease (Xie et al., 2013).

The implications for dementia prevention are significant. Even a single night of sleep deprivation has been shown to increase measurable levels of amyloid-beta in the human brain the following day. Chronic sleep deprivation, over years and decades, is now considered one of the most significant modifiable risk factors for Alzheimer's disease. As Matthew Walker, the neuroscientist and sleep researcher at UC Berkeley, has described it: wakefulness is, in effect, low-level brain damage — and sleep is the nightly sanitation shift that cleans up the damage. It is worth noting that while the glymphatic hypothesis remains an active area of research and some aspects are still being refined, the broader link between sleep disruption and neurodegeneration risk is now robust across many lines of evidence.

REM Sleep: The Emotional and Cognitive Workshop

REM sleep — the dreaming phase — is where the brain performs its emotional and cognitive maintenance. During REM, the brain consolidates procedural and emotional memories, processes the emotional charge of recent experiences, and makes the kind of cross-associative creative connections that underlie insight and innovation. It is during REM sleep that the brain achieves something remarkable: it replays emotionally significant memories, but in an environment virtually free of the stress hormone noradrenaline. This allows the brain to process emotional experiences without re-traumatising, and to gradually reduce the emotional intensity of difficult memories.

The consequences of REM sleep deprivation are significant and often underappreciated. Insufficient REM sleep impairs emotional regulation — you become more reactive, more anxious, and less able to read social cues accurately. It impairs creativity and problem-solving. And over time, it contributes to the cognitive decline and emotional dysregulation that are often attributed simply to ageing.

One of the important findings from sleep research is that both deep NREM and REM sleep are necessary — they cannot substitute for each other. A full night of sleep is needed to complete the natural cycling between stages. This is why sleep architecture matters, not just duration.

What Chronic Poor Sleep Does to Your Body

The research on the consequences of insufficient sleep is, quite frankly, alarming — particularly for a society that has normalised sleeping far less than the recommended seven to nine hours. Let us go through the main consequences, because understanding them is important motivation for taking sleep seriously.

Cardiovascular Disease

A meta-analysis published in GeroScience in 2025, encompassing data from over 79 cohort studies, found that short sleep duration — defined as less than seven hours per night — was associated with a 14 per cent increase in all-cause mortality risk compared to the reference of seven to eight hours. Longer sleep (more than nine hours) was associated with an even greater risk increase of 24 to 34 per cent, likely reflecting underlying illness rather than a causal effect of sleep itself (GeroScience, 2025).

Sleep deprivation elevates blood pressure — both during the day and, critically, at night, when blood pressure would normally fall during the restorative dipping phase. Research from the Mayo Clinic found that even in otherwise healthy people, restricting sleep to four hours per night led to significant rises in blood pressure that persisted even when participants subsequently had the opportunity to sleep deeply. Over time, this sustained elevation contributes to the accelerated cardiovascular ageing seen in short sleepers.

Metabolic Health and Weight

Sleep deprivation disrupts the hormones that regulate appetite — specifically, it suppresses leptin (the satiety hormone) and elevates ghrelin (the hunger hormone). The practical result: sleep-deprived people consume more calories, make poorer food choices, and preferentially store excess energy as visceral fat rather than subcutaneous fat. Research from the Mayo Clinic found that healthy participants sleeping only four hours per night consumed an average of 350 extra calories the following day, and the excess was stored as visceral, inflammation-producing fat.

Chronic sleep deprivation also promotes insulin resistance and impaired glucose tolerance — key drivers of type 2 diabetes and metabolic ageing. The association between poor sleep and metabolic dysfunction runs through multiple mechanisms: elevated cortisol, disrupted circadian regulation of glucose metabolism, increased inflammation, and impaired pancreatic beta-cell function. Given that metabolic dysfunction is one of the most potent accelerators of biological ageing — as we discussed in Chapter One — the sleep-metabolism link has direct and significant implications for healthspan.

Cognitive Function and Dementia Risk

The evidence for sleep's role in cognitive health and dementia prevention has strengthened considerably in recent years. Beyond the glymphatic clearance mechanism described above, poor sleep is associated with accelerated brain ageing, reduced grey matter volume, and impaired hippocampal function. A study in Psychosomatic Medicine published in 2024 found that short sleep duration and insomnia were both associated with accelerated epigenetic ageing — a direct demonstration of the link between sleep deprivation and faster biological ageing at the cellular level (Kusters et al., 2024).

The relationship between sleep and Alzheimer's disease risk is now considered bidirectional: poor sleep accelerates amyloid accumulation, and amyloid accumulation in turn impairs sleep quality — creating a vicious cycle in which sleep disruption accelerates the very pathological process that further disrupts sleep. Intervening on sleep quality, particularly deep sleep, is increasingly regarded as one of the most accessible preventive strategies for neurodegenerative disease.

Immune Function and Cancer Risk

A single night of poor sleep can reduce natural killer cell activity — a key component of the immune system's anti-cancer surveillance — by as much as 70 per cent in some studies. Chronic sleep deprivation is associated with impaired vaccine responses, increased susceptibility to infection, and elevated risk of several cancers. The immune system performs much of its maintenance and memory consolidation during sleep, particularly during the deep NREM stages.

Biological Ageing

At the molecular level, sleep deprivation accelerates virtually every hallmark of ageing. It impairs DNA repair, promotes epigenetic dysregulation, increases cellular senescence, drives inflammation, disrupts nutrient-sensing pathways, and shortens telomeres. A systematic review published in 2019 found that delayed sleep onset was associated with shorter telomere length. As noted above, the 2024 study by Kusters and colleagues confirmed that both short sleep and insomnia are independently associated with accelerated epigenetic ageing.

The 2024 landmark study from Monash University, published in the journal Sleep, added an important dimension: it found that sleep regularity — the day-to-day consistency of your sleep-wake timing — was a stronger predictor of all-cause mortality than sleep duration. People with irregular sleep timing had significantly higher mortality rates even when total sleep time was adequate (Windred et al., 2024). This finding underscores the importance of consistent sleep scheduling as part of a healthspan approach.

"Sleep regularity — going to bed and waking at consistent times — is a stronger predictor of mortality risk than sleep duration alone." — Windred et al., Sleep, 2024

How Much Sleep Do You Actually Need?

The evidence-based recommendation for adults is seven to nine hours of sleep per night. This is not a range with much flexibility at the lower end — the research consistently shows that sleeping less than seven hours on a regular basis is associated with measurably worse health outcomes across virtually every domain.

You may be familiar with people who claim to function perfectly well on five or six hours. For the vast majority, this is not true — it reflects a phenomenon researchers call sleep debt adaptation, in which people lose the ability to accurately perceive their own impairment as sleep deprivation accumulates. They feel fine. They are not fine. Objective tests of cognitive performance, reaction time, and decision-making consistently reveal significant impairment in habitual short sleepers who feel subjectively rested.

There is a small proportion of the population — genuine short sleepers, estimated at less than one per cent — who carry rare genetic variants that allow them to function optimally on six hours or less. Unless you have been genetically tested, the probability that you are one of them is very low.

Age matters too. As we age, sleep architecture changes: deep slow-wave sleep declines, sleep becomes more fragmented, and the ability to obtain restorative sleep requires more attention and care. This is not an excuse to accept poor sleep in later life — it is a reason to prioritise sleep hygiene, identify and treat sleep disorders, and understand that the investment in better sleep yields compounding returns as you age.

Practical Sleep Optimisation: What the Evidence Supports

The good news is that sleep is highly responsive to behavioural intervention. The evidence base for sleep improvement is robust and practical, and most of the most effective strategies cost nothing. Below is a synthesis of what the science consistently supports.

1. Prioritise Sleep Consistency Above All Else

The Monash University finding that sleep regularity predicts mortality more strongly than duration is clinically important. Go to bed and wake up at the same time every day — including weekends. Your circadian rhythm is an internal biological clock that thrives on consistency. Irregular sleep timing disrupts the hormonal and metabolic rhythms that depend on it, even when total sleep time is adequate.

One of the most common mistakes people make is 'catching up' on weekends — sleeping in on Saturday and Sunday to compensate for weekday shortfalls. This social jet lag disrupts the circadian rhythm and compounds rather than resolves the consequences of the weekday sleep deficit.

2. Protect Your Sleep Environment

- Temperature: The optimal bedroom temperature for sleep is cool — around 17 to 19 degrees Celsius. Body temperature needs to drop by approximately one to two degrees to initiate and maintain sleep. A hot bedroom is one of the most common and easily remedied causes of poor sleep quality.

- Darkness: Even small amounts of light can suppress melatonin secretion and disrupt sleep architecture. Blackout curtains or a sleep mask are among the highest-value sleep investments available.

- Quiet: Chronic noise exposure — including traffic and snoring — fragments sleep architecture even when it does not cause full awakenings. Earplugs or a white noise machine can be highly effective.

- Screens: The blue light emitted by phones, tablets, and televisions suppresses melatonin and delays sleep onset. The content itself — stimulating, emotionally activating — has an additional activating effect. The evidence supports removing screens from the bedroom and avoiding them for at least one hour before bed.

3. Manage Light and Darkness Strategically

Light is the most powerful regulator of the circadian clock. Morning sunlight exposure — ideally within thirty to sixty minutes of waking, outdoors, without sunglasses — powerfully anchors your circadian rhythm and improves sleep onset that evening. This is one of the most evidence-supported and underutilised sleep interventions available. For Australians, it also has the advantage of being completely free and widely accessible.

Evening light management is the complementary half. Dimming lights after sunset, using warm-toned lighting indoors, and limiting bright screen exposure in the hours before bed all support the natural rise of melatonin that signals the body to prepare for sleep.

4. Be Cautious with Alcohol and Caffeine

Alcohol is one of the most widely misunderstood sleep disruptors. It does help people fall asleep faster — which is why many people reach for a nightcap. But it dramatically impairs sleep quality: it suppresses REM sleep, fragments sleep architecture in the second half of the night, and increases the frequency of brief arousals that people are often unaware of but that significantly reduce restorative sleep. Drinking alcohol to improve sleep is, in effect, trading sleep onset for sleep quality — a poor exchange.

Caffeine has a half-life of approximately five to seven hours in most people, meaning that a cup of coffee at 3pm will still have roughly half its caffeine content circulating at 8 or 9pm. For those who are sensitive to caffeine or sleeping poorly, moving the cut-off earlier —

no caffeine after noon or 1pm — can produce meaningful improvements in sleep quality.

5. Cognitive Behavioural Therapy for Insomnia (CBT-I)

If you are struggling with chronic insomnia — difficulty falling asleep, staying asleep, or waking too early on a regular basis — the most evidence-based treatment available is Cognitive Behavioural Therapy for Insomnia, or CBT-I. It is recommended as first-line treatment by every major sleep medicine body internationally, including the American Academy of Sleep Medicine, the World Sleep Society, and Australasian Sleep Association guidelines.

CBT-I works by addressing the cognitive patterns (worry and catastrophising about sleep), behavioural patterns (lying awake in bed, variable sleep timing), and physiological patterns (hyperarousal) that perpetuate chronic insomnia. Compared to sleeping medications, CBT-I produces longer-lasting improvements with no side effects and no dependency. A 2024 Australian randomised controlled trial confirmed the effectiveness of digital CBT-I programs for people who cannot access face-to-face therapy — making it more accessible than ever.

In Australia, CBT-I can be accessed through clinical psychologists (via a GP Mental Health Treatment Plan for partial Medicare rebate), online programs such as Sleepio, and a growing number of sleep clinics. If you are relying on sleeping pills for chronic insomnia, please speak with your doctor about a referral for CBT-I — the evidence strongly supports it as a more effective long-term solution.

6. Address Sleep Apnoea

Obstructive sleep apnoea — in which the airway repeatedly collapses during sleep, causing brief arousals that prevent deep, restorative sleep — is estimated to affect at least eight per cent of Australian adults, and many more are undiagnosed. The consequences are significant: untreated OSA is associated with increased risk of cardiovascular disease, metabolic dysfunction, cognitive decline, depression, and all-cause mortality.

If you snore loudly, wake feeling unrefreshed despite adequate time in bed, experience excessive daytime sleepiness, or have been told you stop breathing in your sleep, please speak with your GP about a sleep study referral. Home-based sleep studies are now widely available in Australia and can diagnose OSA without an overnight hospital stay. Either mandibular advancement systems (MAS) or CPAP (Continuous Positive Airway Pressure) therapy can be effective treatment for moderate to severe OSA and can produce dramatic improvements in sleep quality, energy, cognitive function, and long-term health outcomes. CPAP is very effective but poorly tolerated, so compliance is low, whereas MAS are very well tolerated and highly effective.

Sleep and the Hallmarks: Connecting the Science

It is worth pausing to appreciate just how broadly sleep touches the hallmarks of ageing discussed in Chapter One. Sleep is not simply one factor among many — it is the biological foundation on which almost every other health intervention is built.

Hallmark of Ageing	How Sleep Affects It
Genomic instability	DNA repair is completed and consolidated during sleep. Deprivation impairs repair mechanisms, accelerating genomic damage.
Telomere attrition	Short sleep and insomnia are independently associated with shorter telomere length and accelerated epigenetic ageing.
Epigenetic alterations	Sleep deprivation causes measurable epigenetic age acceleration. Good sleep supports epigenetic stability.
Loss of proteostasis	Deep sleep activates protein quality control and clears misfolded proteins via the glymphatic and autophagic systems.
Mitochondrial dysfunction	Sleep supports mitochondrial repair and biogenesis. Chronic deprivation impairs mitochondrial function and energy production.
Cellular senescence	Sleep deprivation accelerates the accumulation of senescent cells by increasing oxidative stress and DNA damage.

Hallmark of Ageing	How Sleep Affects It
Inflammageing	Short sleep consistently elevates CRP, IL-6, and other inflammatory markers. Adequate sleep is one of the most powerful anti-inflammatory interventions.
Dysbiosis	Sleep disruption alters gut microbiome composition, reducing diversity and promoting pro-inflammatory species.
Deregulated nutrient sensing	Sleep deprivation dysregulates insulin, leptin, ghrelin, and cortisol — all critical nutrient-sensing hormones.

The Single Best Investment You Can Make

If I could give every patient I have ever seen one piece of advice — one intervention that would move the needle most on their long-term health — it would be this: protect your sleep.

Not because everything else is less important. Exercise, nutrition, stress management, and connection all matter enormously, as the chapters that follow will make clear. But sleep is the foundation on which all of them rest. When sleep is poor, exercise recovery is impaired. Dietary choices deteriorate. Stress hormones are elevated. Emotional regulation collapses. Biological ageing accelerates across every measurable dimension.

Conversely, when sleep is prioritised and protected, virtually every other aspect of health improves. The research is unambiguous and the investment required is, compared to most things in health, extraordinarily accessible. You do not need a prescription, a gym membership, or a specialist referral. You need a consistent bedtime, a dark and cool bedroom, an early morning walk in the sunlight, and the cultural permission — which this book is explicitly granting you — to take your sleep as seriously as your health demands.

Start tonight.

Chapter Summary

- Sleep is the single most powerful modifiable determinant of healthspan, touching every major biological system and all twelve hallmarks of ageing.

- Around 40 per cent of Australian adults regularly experience inadequate sleep. Inadequate sleep costs the Australian economy an estimated $66.3 billion annually. Most sleep disorders are significantly undertreated.

- Deep NREM sleep drives physical repair, DNA maintenance, hormone secretion, and glymphatic brain clearance. REM sleep supports emotional regulation, memory, and cognitive function. Both are essential.

- Short sleep (under seven hours) is associated with a 14 per cent increase in all-cause mortality. Long sleep (over nine hours) carries a 24–34 per cent increase, likely reflecting underlying illness.

- Sleep regularity — consistent sleep-wake timing — is a stronger predictor of mortality risk than sleep duration alone (Windred et al., 2024).

- Chronic poor sleep accelerates cardiovascular ageing, metabolic dysfunction, cognitive decline, immune suppression, and biological ageing across multiple epigenetic measures.

- Cognitive Behavioural Therapy for Insomnia (CBT-I) is the recommended first-line treatment for chronic insomnia, producing lasting results without the side effects or dependency risks of sleeping medications.

- Key practical interventions: consistent sleep-wake timing, cool dark bedroom, morning sunlight exposure, limiting screens and alcohol before bed, caffeine cut-off before 1pm, and screening for sleep apnoea if symptoms are present.

References

Windred, D. P., Burns, A. C., Lane, J. M., Saxena, R., Rutter, M. K., Cain, S. W., & Phillips, A. J. K. (2024). Sleep regularity is a stronger predictor of mortality risk than sleep duration: A prospective cohort study. Sleep, 47(1), zsad253. https://doi.org/10.1093/sleep/zsad253

Fekete, M., Szarvas, Z., Fazekas-Pongor, V., Feher, A., Csipo, T., Forrai, J., et al. (2025). Imbalanced sleep increases mortality risk by 14–34%: a meta-analysis. GeroScience.   https://doi.org/10.1007/s11357-025-01592-y

Walker, M. P. (2017). Why We Sleep: Unlocking the Power of Sleep and Dreams. Scribner.

Xie, L., Kang, H., Xu, Q., Chen, M. J., Liao, Y., Thiyagarajan, M., et al. (2013). Sleep drives metabolite clearance from the adult brain. Science, 342(6156), 373–377.

Kusters, C. D. J., Klopack, E. T., Crimmins, E. M., Seeman, T. E., Cole, S., & Carroll, J. E. (2024). Short sleep and insomnia are associated with accelerated epigenetic age. Psychosomatic Medicine, 86, 453–462.

Sweetman, A., Reynolds, C., Lack, L., Vakulin, A., Chai-Coetzer, C. L., & Wallace, D. M. (2024). Digital cognitive behavioural therapy for insomnia versus digital sleep education control in an Australian community-based sample: a randomised controlled trial. Internal Medicine Journal. https://doi.org/10.1111/imj.16521

Adams, R., et al. (2017). Sleep education for healthcare providers: Addressing deficient sleep in Australia and New Zealand. Sleep Medicine Reviews, 21, 9–17.

Australasian Sleep Association. (2024). Australasian Sleep Association 2024 guidelines for sleep studies in adults. Sleep, 47(10), zsae107.

Irwin, M. R. (2019). Sleep and inflammation: partners in sickness and in health. Nature Reviews Immunology, 19(11), 702–715.

Cappuccio, F. P., D'Elia, L., Strazzullo, P., & Miller, M. A. (2010). Sleep duration and all-cause mortality: A systematic review and meta-analysis of prospective studies. Sleep, 33(5), 585–592.

Chapter Five

Movement: The Closest Thing to a Longevity Drug

*Why exercise is not just good for you —
it is the most powerful anti-ageing
intervention available*

There is a thought experiment that Peter Attia, the longevity physician, uses to illustrate the power of exercise. He asks: if a pharmaceutical company developed a drug that simultaneously reduced all-cause mortality by 30 to 35 per cent, cut cardiovascular disease risk in half, significantly lowered the risk of type 2 diabetes, cancer, dementia, and depression, improved bone density, preserved muscle mass and strength, enhanced cognitive function, and produced favourable changes in virtually every measurable biomarker of ageing — would you take it? Of course you would. Everyone would.

That drug does not exist. But the effect described is not hypothetical — it is what the evidence consistently shows for regular physical exercise. The meta-analyses are unambiguous. The mechanistic research is compelling. And unlike most pharmaceuticals, the benefits compound over time, improve with consistent use, and have no serious side effects when applied appropriately.

Yet only around 15 per cent of Australian adults meet combined guidelines for both aerobic and strength-based physical activity. We are, as a nation, significantly underutilising the most powerful longevity intervention available to us.

This chapter covers what the science actually shows about exercise and biological ageing — not the superficial 'exercise is good for you' message you have heard a thousand times, but the specific mechanisms, the most effective modes, and the practical framework for building a movement practice that will genuinely change your biological age. We will also address the most common barriers and misconceptions, because understanding why exercise is important is only useful if it translates into actually doing it.

Fitness as a Vital Sign: The VO₂max Story

Of all the measurable physical parameters that predict long-term health outcomes, maximal aerobic capacity — known as VO_2max — stands apart. VO_2max is the maximum rate at which your body can transport and utilise oxygen during exercise. It reflects the integrated performance of your heart, lungs, blood, and muscles — and it is, quite simply, one of the most powerful predictors of mortality and healthspan available.

The evidence is striking. A comprehensive overview of systematic reviews, published in 2024, found that high cardiorespiratory fitness was associated with a 53 per cent lower risk of all-cause mortality compared to low fitness (hazard ratio 0.47). Each one-MET increase in fitness — a modest, achievable improvement — was associated with an 11 to 17 per cent reduction in all-cause mortality. For heart failure specifically, the risk reduction for high versus low fitness was 69 per cent. These are not small effects — they dwarf the mortality benefits of most pharmaceutical interventions.

A landmark 46-year follow-up study of middle-aged men, published in the Journal of the American College of Cardiology, found that each one-unit increase in VO₂max was associated with an additional 45 days of life — and that the benefits of higher midlife fitness extended well into the later decades of life (Loe et al., 2018). The protective effect was not diminished by age, cardiovascular risk factors, or smoking status.

The American Heart Association now recommends that cardiorespiratory fitness be assessed and reported as a clinical vital sign — alongside blood pressure, heart rate, and weight — because of its predictive power for long-term health outcomes. In Australia, VO₂max is assessable through exercise physiologists and increasingly through longevity clinics. For a meaningful proxy, submaximal tests performed by an exercise physiologist, or the Rockport Walk Test, provide useful estimates without the need for a full laboratory assessment.

"High cardiorespiratory fitness is associated with a 53% lower risk of all-cause mortality compared to low fitness — a benefit that dwarfs most pharmaceutical interventions."

The relationship between VO₂max and biological ageing runs through multiple mechanisms: mitochondrial function, cardiovascular efficiency, metabolic health, and the anti-inflammatory effects of regular aerobic training. A 2024 meta-analysis also confirmed that individuals with higher VO₂max have significantly longer telomeres — a direct marker of biological ageing — with the association particularly strong at fitness levels in the 70th percentile or above (Journals of Gerontology, 2024).

What makes this clinically meaningful is that VO$_2$max is highly trainable at any age. You do not need to be an athlete. Moving from the lowest fitness quintile to the second-lowest produces larger mortality benefits than any subsequent step up the fitness ladder. In other words, the gains from going from unfit to moderately fit are the greatest available — and they are available to everyone.

Muscle: The Organ of Longevity

If aerobic fitness is the strongest single predictor of longevity, muscle mass and strength run a very close second. Skeletal muscle is not simply the tissue that moves your body — it is one of the most metabolically active organs you have, performing functions that are central to metabolic health, immune regulation, hormonal balance, and even cognitive function.

Sarcopenia — the progressive loss of muscle mass and function that begins as early as the mid-thirties and accelerates after 60 — is one of the most significant and underappreciated drivers of poor healthspan. It is associated with increased risk of falls and fractures, metabolic dysfunction, insulin resistance, cognitive decline, depression, loss of independence, and all-cause mortality. Grip strength — one of the simplest proxies for overall muscle function — is a more powerful predictor of cardiovascular mortality than systolic blood pressure in some analyses.

The good news is that muscle loss is not inevitable. It is strongly modifiable through resistance training —

and the evidence shows that meaningful muscle preservation and even gains are achievable at virtually any age. A systematic review and meta-analysis published in 2022 confirmed that resistance training is associated with significantly reduced risk of all-cause mortality, cardiovascular mortality, and cancer-specific mortality across large populations (Shailendra et al., 2022).

Why Muscle Matters Beyond Movement

Muscle tissue is now understood to function as an endocrine organ — one that communicates with virtually every other organ in the body through signalling molecules called myokines. When muscle contracts during exercise, it releases over 600 different myokines into the circulation. These molecules travel to the brain, liver, fat tissue, bone, immune system, and beyond, exerting effects that go far beyond the muscle itself.

Among the most important myokines for healthspan are Brain-Derived Neurotrophic Factor (BDNF) — often described as fertiliser for the brain — which promotes neurogenesis, synaptic plasticity, and protection against neurodegenerative disease. Irisin, released during muscle contraction, promotes the conversion of metabolically inactive white fat to more active brown fat, improves insulin sensitivity, and crosses the blood-brain barrier to enhance cognitive function. Interleukin-6 (IL-6), released acutely during exercise, acts as a potent anti-inflammatory signal — an important distinction from the chronically elevated IL-6 seen in sedentary people, which drives the inflammageing discussed in Chapter One (Pedersen & Febbraio, 2012).

In practical terms: every time you exercise, your muscles release a cascade of beneficial molecular signals that improve your brain, your metabolism, your immune system, and your bones — simultaneously. The muscle is not just doing work. It is communicating.

The Three Pillars of Movement for Healthspan

The evidence supports a three-pillar approach to movement for long-term health: aerobic training (with both Zone 2 and higher-intensity components), resistance training, and mobility and balance work. Each serves distinct functions. Together, they constitute a comprehensive, evidence-based movement practice for healthspan.

Pillar 1: Aerobic Training — Zone 2 and High Intensity

Aerobic exercise — any sustained rhythmic activity that elevates heart rate and breathing — is the primary driver of cardiovascular fitness, mitochondrial health, and VO_2max. For healthspan purposes, the evidence supports training across two key intensity zones.

Zone 2 training — sustained moderate-intensity exercise at roughly 60 to 70 per cent of maximum heart rate, where you can hold a conversation but are working steadily — is the foundation. It is the primary stimulus for mitochondrial biogenesis (the creation of new, functional mitochondria), fat oxidation, and long-term cardiovascular adaptation. Zone 2 builds the aerobic base that underpins everything else. Research by exercise physiologist Dr Iñigo San-Millán has shown that elite endurance athletes spend around 80 per cent of their training time in Zone 2 — a principle that translates well to the general population seeking health and longevity. The recommendation is a minimum of 150 to 180 minutes of Zone 2 per week, achievable through brisk walking, cycling, swimming, rowing, or any activity that keeps you in the moderate effort range.

High-intensity interval training (HIIT) — shorter bursts of near-maximal effort followed by recovery periods — is the most time-efficient way to improve VO_2max and stimulate mitochondrial adaptation. A typical HIIT protocol of one to two sessions per week, each lasting 20 to 30 minutes, provides a powerful stimulus that complements the Zone 2 base. Research published in the European Journal of Preventive Cardiology in 2025 found that exercise intensity was a primary driver of mortality risk reduction, suggesting that including some higher-intensity work may be particularly valuable for longevity. A practical approach for most people is 80 per cent of aerobic time in Zone 2 and approximately 20 per cent in higher-intensity zones.

Pillar 2: Resistance Training

Resistance training — any exercise that challenges muscles against a load, whether that is free weights, machines, resistance bands, or bodyweight — is the primary driver of muscle mass preservation, bone density, and metabolic health. It is the non-negotiable second pillar of a healthspan-focused movement practice.

The current Australian Physical Activity Guidelines recommend at least two days of muscle-strengthening activity per week for adults, and this should be considered a minimum rather than an optimal target.

For most middle-aged and older adults pursuing healthspan, three sessions per week — targeting all major muscle groups — is a practical and effective approach. The key principles are progressive overload (gradually increasing challenge over time), consistency, and attention to compound movements that load multiple muscle groups simultaneously: squats, deadlifts, rows, presses, and their variations.

A 2025 systematic review and meta-analysis found that resistance training significantly improved muscle strength and physical function in older adults with sarcopenia — with meaningful, clinically relevant effect sizes even in those with established muscle loss. Critically, resistance training benefits are not age-limited. Studies in adults in their 70s, 80s, and beyond consistently demonstrate significant strength and muscle gains in response to progressive resistance training.

For bone health specifically, the evidence is compelling. A series of trials from Edith Cowan University in Australia — including the landmark LIFTMOR trials led by Dr Belinda Beck — demonstrated that supervised high-intensity resistance and impact training significantly increased lumbar spine bone mineral density in postmenopausal women with osteopenia and osteoporosis, and did so safely. This directly addresses one of the most consequential age-related declines: the bone fragility that leads to fractures, hospitalisation, and loss of independence.

Pillar 3: Mobility, Balance, and Functional Movement

The third pillar is less discussed but increasingly recognised as critical for long-term functional independence: mobility, balance, and the ability to move well through daily life. Falls are one of the most devastating events in older adult health — over 380,000 older Australians are hospitalised due to falls each year, with consequences ranging from fracture and disability to death. The ability to maintain balance, move with confidence, and recover from perturbation is a trainable physical quality that declines rapidly with age and inactivity.

Exercise and Sports Science Australia (ESSA) released an updated position statement in 2024 recommending that falls prevention exercise for community-dwelling older Australians should include challenging balance training as a core component — not just strength work. Activities such as single-leg exercises, balance board training, tai chi, yoga, and functional movement patterns all contribute to this capacity.

A simple and clinically meaningful test: can you stand on one leg for ten seconds with your eyes open? Research published in the British Journal of Sports Medicine found that the inability to perform this test was associated with nearly twice the risk of all-cause mortality over a ten-year follow-up period in middle-aged and older adults. This is not a party trick — it is a meaningful indicator of neuromuscular ageing and fall risk.

A Practical Weekly Movement Framework

One of the most common barriers to exercise is not motivation — it is not knowing what to actually do, or feeling overwhelmed by conflicting advice. The following framework is drawn directly from the evidence and is designed to be realistic for a busy working adult. It is a starting point, not a prescription — individual needs, capacity, and starting points vary.

Day	Activity	Notes
Monday	Resistance training — lower body focus (30–45 min)	Squats, deadlifts, leg press, calf raises. Progressive load.
Tuesday	Zone 2 aerobic (45–60 min)	Brisk walk, cycle, swim, or row. Conversational pace.
Wednesday	Resistance training — upper body focus (30–45 min)	Push/pull movements: rows, presses, lat pulldowns. Add core.
Thursday	Zone 2 aerobic + mobility (45 min)	Aerobic session followed by 10–15 min stretching/mobility work.
Friday	Resistance training — full body or weak areas (30–45 min)	Focus on areas needing attention. Include single-leg balance work.
Saturday	HIIT or higher-intensity aerobic (20–30 min)	Interval session: 4–8 hard efforts of 3–4 min with equal recovery.
Sunday	Active recovery / incidental movement	Walk, gentle yoga, or simply stay off the couch. Rest is valid.

This is a template, not a mandate. Three days of exercise is substantially better than none. Two is better than one. The most important exercise principle for healthspan is consistency over time — not perfection in any single week. If the above feels like too much, start with two resistance sessions and two to three walks per week and build from there.

Starting from Scratch: What to Do if You Are Currently Inactive

The research on exercise and mortality is particularly empowering for those who are currently doing very little. The largest mortality benefit from exercise accrues when sedentary individuals begin any regular movement — even modest amounts. Moving from the least fit quintile to the second-least fit produces a larger reduction in mortality risk than any subsequent improvement.

If you are currently largely sedentary, the evidence strongly supports starting with walking. It is accessible, low-injury-risk, requires no equipment, and produces measurable improvements in cardiovascular fitness, metabolic health, and psychological wellbeing. A daily 30-minute brisk walk — defined as a pace where you feel slightly breathless but can still hold a conversation — is a legitimate and meaningful intervention. It is not the ceiling of what is possible, but it is an excellent and evidence-based starting point.

Adding two sessions of resistance training per week — even bodyweight exercises at home — is the next step. Squats, lunges, push-ups, and rows performed consistently will produce meaningful gains in strength and muscle preservation. Starting with a qualified exercise physiologist is highly recommended for anyone over 50, anyone with existing musculoskeletal issues, or anyone who has been sedentary for an extended period. In Australia, exercise physiologists can be accessed through a GP Chronic Disease Management plan with a partial Medicare rebate.

The principle of progressive overload is important from the beginning. This means gradually and consistently increasing the challenge — either the weight lifted, the duration of exercise, the intensity, or some combination — over weeks and months. The body adapts to the demands placed on it. Consistent moderate challenge produces consistent improvement. Staying at the same level indefinitely produces a plateau.

Exercise and the Hallmarks of Ageing

As we discussed in Chapter One, the hallmarks of ageing are twelve interconnected biological processes that drive cellular and tissue decline. Exercise is arguably the most broadly effective intervention we have for addressing multiple hallmarks simultaneously — a key reason why its effects on mortality and healthspan are so large.

Hallmark	How Exercise Addresses It
Genomic instability	Exercise upregulates DNA repair enzymes and reduces oxidative DNA damage.
Telomere attrition	Higher VO_2max and regular aerobic exercise are independently associated with longer telomeres.

Hallmark	How Exercise Addresses It
Epigenetic alterations	Exercise produces favourable epigenetic changes including reduced biological age on methylation clocks.
Mitochondrial dysfunction	Aerobic and interval training are the most potent known stimuli for mitochondrial biogenesis.
Cellular senescence	Exercise reduces the burden of senescent cells and promotes their clearance by the immune system.
Inflammageing	Myokines released during exercise have potent anti-inflammatory effects; regular training reduces hsCRP and IL-6.
Stem cell exhaustion	Resistance training stimulates muscle stem cell (satellite cell) activity; exercise preserves bone marrow stem cell function.
Dysbiosis	Regular exercise promotes gut microbiome diversity and reduces dysbiosis.
Loss of proteostasis	Exercise activates autophagy and the cellular protein quality control systems.
Deregulated nutrient sensing	Exercise activates AMPK and modulates mTOR and insulin signalling pathways beneficially.

Common Barriers and How to Address Them

"I am too busy."

The minimum effective dose for significant health benefits — two resistance sessions and 150 minutes of moderate aerobic activity per week — requires roughly four to five hours. That is less than four per cent of your waking hours. Research consistently shows that the time investment in exercise pays returns in energy, productivity, and cognitive function that far exceed the time spent. HIIT protocols can deliver meaningful cardiovascular benefit in as little as 20 minutes. Brief resistance training sessions of 30 minutes, performed consistently, produce real results.

"I am too old to start."

There is no age at which the benefits of exercise disappear. Studies in adults in their eighties and nineties consistently demonstrate significant strength, muscle, and functional gains in response to resistance training. Frailty is not an inevitable consequence of age — in many cases, it is a consequence of inactivity. The appropriate question is not whether to start, but how to start safely — which is where an exercise physiologist can be invaluable.

"I have a bad knee / back / shoulder."

Chronic pain and musculoskeletal issues are common barriers, and they are often self-reinforcing: inactivity leads to muscle weakness, which worsens joint loading and pain, which leads to more inactivity. The answer for most people is not to avoid exercise but to find the right exercise — usually guided by an exercise physiologist or physiotherapist who can design a programme that works around and progressively rehabilitates the affected area. Exercise is now recommended as a first-line intervention for most forms of chronic musculoskeletal pain, including osteoarthritis.

"I already do enough walking."

Walking is excellent and should absolutely be part of a healthspan-focused movement practice. But it does not preserve muscle mass, build bone density, or adequately stress the cardiovascular system for the most significant longevity benefits. It is the floor, not the ceiling. The evidence supports walking plus resistance training plus occasional higher-intensity aerobic work — not walking alone.

Movement Is Medicine

There is no supplement, no diet, no emerging therapeutic that approaches the breadth, robustness, and magnitude of the evidence for regular physical exercise as a longevity intervention. It is the single most impactful thing most people can do to improve their biological age, reduce their chronic disease risk, preserve cognitive function, and extend their healthspan.

The barriers are real — time, energy, injury, knowledge, and the sheer inertia of established sedentary habits. But the evidence is also clear that very modest amounts of movement, applied consistently, produce substantial benefits. The goal is not to become an athlete. It is to become someone who moves regularly, challenges their muscles two to three times per week, does enough aerobic work to maintain a meaningful level of cardiovascular fitness, and takes their physical capacity seriously as a long-term asset.

Start with what you can manage. Build from there. And remember: the compounding effect of consistent movement over years and decades is the real prize. Every session is an investment in the person you will be at 70, 80, and beyond.

Chapter Summary

- Regular physical exercise reduces all-cause mortality by 30 to 35 per cent compared to inactivity — an effect that exceeds virtually every pharmaceutical intervention available.

- VO_2max is the single strongest modifiable predictor of longevity. High cardiorespiratory fitness is associated with a 53 per cent lower risk of all-cause mortality. Each one-MET improvement reduces mortality risk by 11–17 per cent.

- Muscle mass and strength are independently associated with reduced mortality, better metabolic health, and preserved cognitive function. Sarcopenia is a major and underappreciated driver of poor healthspan.

- Skeletal muscle is an endocrine organ that releases myokines — signalling molecules that benefit the brain (BDNF), metabolism (irisin, IL-6), immune system, and bone — with every contraction.

- A comprehensive movement practice for healthspan requires three pillars: aerobic training (Zone 2 and higher intensity), resistance training, and mobility and balance work.

- The minimum effective target is 150–180 minutes of moderate aerobic activity and two to three resistance training sessions per week. Starting from inactivity produces the largest marginal benefit.

- Exercise addresses ten of the twelve hallmarks of ageing simultaneously — making it the most broadly effective anti-ageing intervention known.

- Exercise physiologists can be accessed in Australia via a GP Chronic Disease Management plan (partial Medicare rebate) and are especially recommended for those starting from inactivity or with existing health conditions.

References

Strain, T., et al. (2024). Cardiorespiratory fitness and health outcomes: An overview of systematic reviews. British Journal of Sports Medicine. https://doi.org/10.1136/bjsports-2023-106746

Loe, H., Steinshamn, S., & Wisløff, U. (2018). Midlife cardiorespiratory fitness and the long-term risk of mortality: 46 years of follow-up. Journal of the American College of Cardiology. https://doi.org/10.1016/j.jacc.2018.06.045

Shailendra, P., Baldock, K. L., Li, L. S. K., Boyle, T., & Bennie, J. A. (2022). Resistance training and mortality risk: A systematic review and meta-analysis. American Journal of Preventive Medicine, 63(2), 277–285.

Pedersen, B. K., & Febbraio, M. A. (2012). Muscles, exercise and obesity: skeletal muscle as a secretory organ. Nature Reviews Endocrinology, 8(8), 457–465.

Schwendinger, F., et al. (2025). Intensity or volume: the role of physical activity in longevity. European Journal of Preventive Cardiology, 32(1), 10–19.

Sherrington, C., et al. (2024). Exercise and Sports Science Australia updated position statement on exercise for preventing falls in older people living in the community. Journal of Science and Medicine in Sport.

Beck, B. R. (2018). High-intensity resistance and impact training improves bone mineral density and physical function in postmenopausal women with osteopenia and osteoporosis: the LIFTMOR randomised controlled trial. Journal of Bone and Mineral Research, 33(2), 211–220.

Zare, H., et al. (2025). Exercise intensity matters: A review on evaluating the effects of aerobic exercise intensity on muscle-derived neuroprotective myokines. Alzheimer's & Dementia: Translational Research & Clinical Interventions. https://doi.org/10.1002/trc2.70056

Gomes-Osman, J., et al. (2024). Systematic review and meta-analysis highlights a link between aerobic fitness and telomere maintenance. Journals of Gerontology Series A, 80(6), glaf068.

Claussen, H. S., & Sherrington, C. (2024). Australian Physical Activity and Sedentary Behaviour Guidelines. Department of Health and Aged Care, Australian Government.

Chapter Six

Nutrition: Evidence-Based Eating for Healthspan

Not another diet — a practical framework for eating in a way that genuinely supports how long and how well you live

---

The nutrition space is, frankly, a mess. For every study supporting a particular dietary approach, there appears to be another one contradicting it. Advocates of high-fat diets argue with proponents of plant-based eating. Intermittent fasting is promoted as transformative by some researchers and dismissed by others. Protein is simultaneously described as essential for longevity and dangerous for kidneys. Carbohydrates are demonised, rehabilitated, and demonised again.

This noise is genuinely confusing for people who simply want to know what to eat. And it has had a real effect: in the absence of clear guidance, many people default either to the last thing they read, the most extreme thing they have tried, or the familiar comfort of habits that are not serving them.

Here is the thing that tends to get lost in the polarised debate: the evidence base for nutrition and longevity, while imperfect, is not as contradictory as it appears. When you look across the large bodies of observational and interventional research — across populations, dietary patterns, and biological mechanisms — a coherent picture emerges. It does not involve a specific named diet. It does not require eliminating entire food groups. And it does not demand perfection.

This chapter will give you that picture: what the science most consistently supports, what the major threats to your healthspan are from a dietary perspective, and how to build a practical eating approach that works in the real world — including the Australian food environment.

The Most Studied Dietary Pattern in the World: Mediterranean Eating

Of all the dietary patterns examined in longevity research, the Mediterranean dietary pattern has accumulated the most robust and consistent evidence base. This is not because Mediterranean food is inherently magical or because olive oil contains some secret compound that other oils do not. It is because this pattern of eating has been studied in large populations over long time periods, and the findings hold up remarkably well across different study designs, populations, and analytical approaches.

A 2024 meta-analysis published in JAMA Network Open, following 25,315 women for 25 years, found that high adherence to the Mediterranean diet was associated with a 23 per cent reduced risk of all-cause mortality. The authors found that this benefit was mediated through improvements in inflammatory markers, triglyceride-rich lipoproteins, insulin resistance, and body composition — not simply through the well-known effects on cholesterol (Ahmad et al., 2024).

A second meta-analysis published in Nutrients in 2024, examining 679,259 participants across 28 studies including randomised controlled trials, found that high adherence to the Mediterranean diet reduced all-cause mortality risk by 23 per cent in older adults, and also significantly reduced the risk of cardiovascular events (Furbatto et al., 2024). A separate review of randomised controlled trials found that Mediterranean diet adherence was associated with a 48 per cent reduction in major adverse cardiovascular events compared to control diets.

"High adherence to the Mediterranean diet is consistently associated with a 23% reduction in all-cause mortality — mediated through reductions in inflammation, metabolic dysfunction, and cardiovascular risk."

What does the Mediterranean dietary pattern actually look like? It is not a rigid prescription. It is a pattern characterised by an abundance of: vegetables, legumes, whole grains, fruits, nuts, and seeds; olive oil as the primary fat; fish and seafood eaten regularly; poultry, eggs, and dairy in moderate amounts; red meat eaten infrequently; and a general cultural emphasis on whole, minimally processed foods prepared and shared in social contexts.

The good news for Australians is that this pattern maps very well onto what is available here. Fresh vegetables, legumes, fish, olive oil, and seasonal fruit are accessible and affordable across most of the country. The Mediterranean diet is not exotic or expensive — it is primarily a matter of prioritising whole foods over processed ones, and building meals around plant foods rather than treating them as an afterthought.

The Single Greatest Dietary Threat to Your Healthspan: Ultra-Processed Foods

If the Mediterranean dietary pattern represents the positive end of the dietary evidence spectrum, ultra-processed foods (UPFs) sit firmly at the negative end — and the strength of the evidence against them has grown considerably in recent years.

Ultra-processed foods are defined by the NOVA food classification system as industrially manufactured products that contain ingredients rarely used in home cooking — emulsifiers, thickeners, artificial flavours, colours, sweeteners, and preservatives — and which have typically been engineered to be hyper-palatable, calorie-dense, and highly convenient. They include commercially produced breads, packaged snacks, sugary drinks, reconstituted meat products, instant noodles, mass-produced pastries, and most fast food.

A landmark 2024 umbrella review published in the BMJ, examining data from nearly ten million participants across 45 meta-analyses, found direct associations between UPF consumption and 32 adverse health outcomes. These spanned mortality, cancer, cardiovascular disease, metabolic health, respiratory conditions, gastrointestinal disease, and mental health outcomes. The highest level of evidence — classified as 'convincing' — supported associations with cardiovascular disease mortality and type 2 diabetes (Lane et al., 2024).

A 2025 updated systematic review and meta-analysis, combining 18 cohort studies with over 1.1 million participants and 173,000 deaths, found that the highest UPF consumers had a 15 per cent increased risk of all-cause mortality compared to the lowest consumers, with every 10 per cent increment in UPF consumption associated with a further 10 per cent increase in mortality risk.

The mechanisms driving these associations are multiple and mutually reinforcing. Ultra-processed foods are typically high in refined carbohydrates, added sugars, industrial seed oils, and sodium while being low in fibre, micronutrients, and health-protective phytochemicals. They drive dysbiosis by starving beneficial gut bacteria of fibre while feeding pathogenic species. They promote inflammation through their additive profiles and nutrient composition. They disrupt appetite regulation by overriding normal satiety signals, leading to overconsumption. They deliver caloric density without the structural complexity that whole foods use to slow absorption and promote satiety.

In Australia — as in most high-income countries — ultra-processed foods now account for a large share of daily energy intake. Research suggests that in some demographic groups, UPFs may represent over 40 per cent of total energy consumption. This is not simply a matter of individual choice: these products are aggressively marketed, engineered for addictive eating patterns, widely available, cheaper per calorie than whole foods, and embedded in almost every social eating context. Reducing UPF consumption is one of the highest-yield nutritional interventions available —

and one that does not require following a specific dietary philosophy.

> **23%** reduction in all-cause mortality associated with high Mediterranean diet adherence (Ahmad et al., JAMA Network Open, 2024)
>
> **15%** increased risk of all-cause mortality associated with highest ultra-processed food consumption
>
> **32** adverse health outcomes directly associated with UPF exposure in a 2024 umbrella review of 9.9M participants
>
> **1.2g/kg** minimum protein intake per day recommended for older adults to preserve muscle mass (ESPEN guidelines)

Protein: The Most Underrated Nutritional Issue for Ageing Australians

One of the most consistent findings in nutritional gerontology — the science of how nutrition affects ageing — is that the standard recommendation for protein intake is insufficient for most middle-aged and older adults. Australia's official Nutrient Reference Values (NRVs), published by the NHMRC in 2006, set the RDI for protein at 0.75 to 0.84 grams per kilogram per day for adults. These figures were designed to prevent deficiency in the general population and have not yet been formally updated — though a rolling NRV review is currently underway with updated values anticipated in 2026. In the interim, the clinical and research evidence has moved well ahead of the official figures. For people over 50, and particularly over 65, multiple expert bodies and meta-analyses now clearly support a meaningfully higher target.

As we age, skeletal muscle becomes progressively less sensitive to the anabolic (muscle-building) signal of dietary protein — a phenomenon called anabolic resistance. Simply put, older adults need more protein to stimulate the same degree of muscle protein synthesis as younger people. The consequence of chronic protein insufficiency in the context of this anabolic resistance is accelerated muscle loss, contributing directly to sarcopenia, frailty, metabolic dysfunction, and the cascade of health decline that comes with them.

The European Society for Clinical Nutrition and Metabolism (ESPEN) Expert Group recommends that healthy older people consume at least **1.0 to 1.2 grams of protein per kilogram of body weight per day**, with higher targets — 1.2 to 1.5 grams per kilogram — for those who are malnourished, recovering from illness, or dealing with chronic conditions (Deutz et al., 2014). Multiple subsequent analyses have supported these figures, with some researchers advocating for targets as high as 1.6 grams per kilogram per day during periods of active resistance training.

To put this in practical terms: a 70-kilogram person aiming for 1.2 grams per kilogram per day needs approximately 84 grams of protein daily, rising to around 112 grams at 1.6 grams per kilogram. Both figures are meaningfully higher than what the 2006 Australian NRVs suggest, and substantially higher than what most Australians over 50 are currently consuming. Meeting these targets requires deliberate attention to protein-rich foods at each meal.

Protein Distribution Matters

Beyond total daily protein intake, the distribution across meals appears to matter. Maximising muscle protein synthesis requires reaching a threshold dose of essential amino acids at each meal — research suggests approximately 25 to 40 grams of high-quality protein per meal for older adults. A common pattern in which people consume very little protein at breakfast, a moderate amount at lunch, and a large amount at dinner is suboptimal for muscle preservation. Spreading protein more evenly across meals, with at least 25 to 30 grams of protein at each eating occasion, appears to be more effective for maintaining muscle mass.

Protein Quality

Protein quality — specifically the content of essential amino acids, and in particular leucine, which is the primary trigger for muscle protein synthesis — matters alongside quantity. Animal proteins (meat, fish, eggs, dairy) generally have a more complete essential amino acid profile and are more effectively utilised for muscle synthesis than most plant proteins. This does not mean plant proteins are without value — legumes, tofu, tempeh, edamame, and high-protein grains all contribute meaningfully to protein intake. But for older adults specifically, attention to protein quality and leucine content is worth keeping in mind, particularly for those following primarily plant-based diets.

Key Dietary Principles for Healthspan

Beyond the Mediterranean pattern, the protein evidence, and the UPF threat, there are several specific dietary areas with strong enough evidence to warrant direct mention.

Omega-3 Fatty Acids

Long-chain omega-3 fatty acids — EPA and DHA, found predominantly in oily fish — have a well-established evidence base for cardiovascular protection, anti-inflammatory effects, cognitive preservation, and support for telomere length maintenance. The evidence supports consuming oily fish (salmon, sardines, mackerel, herring, tuna) at least two to three times per week. For those who do not regularly eat fish, high-quality fish oil supplementation (providing 1 to 2 grams of combined EPA and DHA per day) is a reasonable option, though whole food sources are generally preferred where accessible.

Fibre and Polyphenols

Dietary fibre is among the most consistently health-protective nutrients in the evidence base. It feeds beneficial gut bacteria, reduces inflammation, improves lipid and glucose profiles, and is associated with reduced risk of cardiovascular disease, type 2 diabetes, colorectal cancer, and all-cause mortality. Most Australians consume well below the recommended 25 to 30 grams per day. Practical sources include vegetables, legumes, whole grains, nuts, seeds, and fruit.

Polyphenols — the bioactive plant compounds found in colourful vegetables and fruits, green tea, olive oil, dark chocolate, coffee, and red wine — have extensive evidence for anti-inflammatory, antioxidant, and anti-ageing effects at the cellular level. They support the gut microbiome, reduce oxidative stress, and modulate gene expression in ways consistent with improved healthspan. The practical message: eat a wide variety of colourful plant foods. Diversity of plant intake is associated with greater gut microbiome diversity, which is in turn associated with better health outcomes.

Blood Sugar Management

The relationship between dietary carbohydrate quality, blood glucose regulation, and ageing is one of the most clinically important areas of nutritional science. Chronically elevated blood glucose and insulin resistance — driven largely by diets high in refined carbohydrates and added sugars — are among the most potent drivers of accelerated biological ageing, cardiovascular disease, type 2 diabetes, and cognitive decline.

This does not mean eliminating carbohydrates. Whole food carbohydrate sources — legumes, vegetables, intact whole grains, and fruit — are consistent components of healthy dietary patterns worldwide. What the evidence argues against is the chronic consumption of rapidly absorbed refined carbohydrates and added sugars: white bread, sugary drinks, pastries, and the carbohydrate fraction of most ultra-processed foods.

Practical strategies for managing blood sugar through diet include prioritising low-glycaemic-index carbohydrate sources, pairing carbohydrates with protein, fat, and fibre at each meal (which slows glucose absorption), avoiding high-carbohydrate meals without balancing macronutrients, and being mindful of liquid carbohydrates — which bypass many of the satiety mechanisms that solid food engages.

Hydration

Chronic mild dehydration is common in older adults and has measurable effects on cognitive function, energy levels, kidney function, and metabolic health. Thirst sensation declines with age, meaning that by the time an older person feels thirsty, they are often already meaningfully dehydrated. A practical rule of thumb is to aim for pale yellow urine throughout the day — a simple and reliable indicator of adequate hydration. Most adults need approximately 1.5 to 2.5 litres of fluid per day, with more required in hot weather or during physical activity.

Intermittent Fasting and Time-Restricted Eating: What the Evidence Shows

Few nutritional topics have attracted more popular interest — or more overblown claims — in recent years than intermittent fasting. The science is genuinely interesting, but deserves honest treatment.

The biological rationale for fasting protocols is strong. Periods without food intake activate autophagy — the cellular recycling process that clears damaged proteins and organelles, and which we discussed as a hallmark of ageing in Chapter One. Fasting also lowers insulin levels, improves insulin sensitivity, activates AMPK (a key nutrient-sensing pathway associated with longevity), and provides a period of metabolic rest that contrasts with the chronic overstimulation of nutrient-sensing pathways that characterises modern eating patterns.

The most studied fasting approach is time-restricted eating (TRE) — limiting food intake to a specific window of hours each day, typically eight to twelve hours, and fasting for the remainder. A 10:14 or 12:12 pattern (ten to twelve hours of eating, twelve to fourteen hours of fasting) is a practical starting point that is achievable by most people and aligns reasonably well with circadian biology.

The evidence for TRE in humans is promising but still maturing. Most trials to date are relatively short-term and small in scale. The benefits seen consistently include modest improvements in metabolic health markers, reduced inflammation, and in some studies, improvements in body composition. Whether these translate into long-term mortality benefits in humans — as has been demonstrated compellingly in animal models — remains to be established through larger and longer trials.

There is also an important caveat for older adults: fasting protocols that significantly restrict total daily caloric intake can accelerate muscle loss, particularly if protein intake is not carefully maintained on eating days. For people over 60, the muscle-preservation priority means that any fasting protocol should be designed to ensure adequate total protein and calorie intake within the eating window, combined with resistance training. Fasting without attention to protein and muscle is a poor trade-off for most older adults.

My clinical recommendation: if time-restricted eating appeals to you and fits your lifestyle, a 12:12 or 10:14 pattern — essentially stopping eating after an early dinner and not eating again until mid-morning the next day — is a reasonable, low-risk approach that is consistent with the biological rationale. It does not need to be extreme to be effective. More aggressive protocols (OMAD, extended fasting) carry greater risks for older adults and should be approached with care and ideally with clinical guidance.

A Practical Nutritional Framework for Healthspan

Drawing the evidence together, the following principles form a coherent, practical, and evidence-supported nutritional framework for healthspan. This is not a diet programme. It is a set of principles that can be applied flexibly across different food cultures, budgets, and preferences.

Principle	What It Means in Practice
1. Prioritise whole foods	Cook from scratch more than you eat from packets. If a food has a long ingredient list with names you don't recognise, it's likely ultra-processed.
2. Build meals around plants	Half your plate at most meals should be vegetables, legumes, or whole grains. Colour and variety matter.
3. Meet your protein target	Aim for 1.2–1.6g per kilogram of body weight per day. Spread across meals. Include a quality protein source at every eating occasion.
4. Minimise ultra-processed foods	Reduce commercially produced snack foods, sugary drinks, packaged meals, and fast food. Not perfectly — practically.
5. Choose quality fats	Olive oil as your primary cooking and dressing oil. Regular oily fish. Nuts, seeds, avocado. Minimise industrial seed oils and trans fats.

Principle	What It Means in Practice
6. Manage carbohydrate quality	Prefer legumes, intact whole grains, and vegetables over refined carbohydrates. Pair carbs with protein and fat.
7. Eat adequate fibre	25–30g per day from vegetables, legumes, whole grains, nuts, and fruit. Most Australians fall well short.
8. Stay well hydrated	Aim for pale yellow urine. Drink water as your primary beverage. Limit sugary drinks and excessive alcohol.
9. Consider eating timing	A natural 12-hour fasting window overnight (e.g. 7pm to 7am) supports metabolic health and aligns with circadian biology.
10. Eat with others when possible	Social eating is one of the most consistent features of long-lived populations worldwide. The context of food matters.

Navigating the Dietary Wars: An Honest Assessment

No chapter on nutrition would be complete without acknowledging the genuine debates that continue within the evidence base.

Plant-based versus animal foods

The evidence does not support either extreme position. Long-lived populations worldwide eat diets that vary considerably in their animal food content — from the relatively meat-rich Sardinian diet to the predominantly plant-based Okinawan pattern. What long-lived populations consistently share is high consumption of whole, minimally processed plant foods, low consumption of ultra-processed products, and moderate total caloric intake. The evidence supports reducing red meat consumption (particularly processed meat) and increasing legume and vegetable intake. It does not support eliminating all animal foods as a universal healthspan strategy.

The protein debate

The tension between high-protein diets for muscle preservation and concerns about mTOR activation and longevity is genuine. Some researchers, drawing on animal models, argue that protein restriction extends lifespan. Others, drawing on human data, argue that protein insufficiency in older adults accelerates sarcopenia and is the greater risk. The current evidence in humans most consistently supports adequate-to-higher protein intake (1.2 to 1.6 grams per kilogram per day) for people over 50, combined with resistance training. The mTOR concerns are more relevant to younger adults and may be addressed by incorporating periods of lower protein intake (consistent with intermittent fasting) rather than chronic restriction.

Organic versus conventional

The evidence for meaningful health benefits of organic versus conventionally grown food, in terms of long-term health outcomes, is limited. Eating a wide variety of conventionally grown vegetables is considerably more beneficial for most people than eating a narrow range of organic ones. Washing produce thoroughly, avoiding excessive reliance on a small number of pesticide-heavy items, and prioritising whole food intake overall are practical middle positions.

Supplements: What Is Worth Considering?

This book takes a food-first approach to nutrition — for good reason. The evidence base for whole dietary patterns is far more robust than the evidence for any individual supplement, and supplements cannot compensate for a poor dietary foundation. That said, several supplements have sufficient evidence to warrant consideration for specific contexts.

Supplement	Evidence Summary	Who Might Consider It
Vitamin D	Strong evidence for bone health, immune function, and muscle function. Deficiency very common in Australians — paradoxically, despite sunshine.	Anyone with low sun exposure, darker skin, over 70, or documented deficiency (check blood levels first).
Omega-3 (EPA/DHA)	Strong evidence for cardiovascular protection, anti-inflammatory effects, cognitive support.	Those who do not regularly eat oily fish (2–3 serves per week).
Magnesium	Widely deficient in Western populations. Involved in over 300 enzymatic reactions. May support sleep, glucose metabolism, and muscle function.	Adults with poor dietary intake, sleep issues, or high stress. Forms: glycinate or malate preferred.

Supplement	Evidence Summary	Who Might Consider It
Creatine	Strong evidence for muscle strength and mass preservation in older adults, particularly combined with resistance training. Also showing cognitive benefit.	Adults over 50 engaging in resistance training. Particularly valuable for women.
B12	Absorption declines with age due to reduced stomach acid. Deficiency causes neurological and haematological problems.	Adults over 60, those on metformin (which reduces B12 absorption), and those following plant-based diets.

Always discuss supplementation with your GP or a qualified healthcare practitioner before starting, and prioritise blood testing to identify actual deficiencies rather than supplementing blindly. In Australia, vitamin D, B12, magnesium, and iron can all be checked through a standard blood panel.

Food Is Information

One of the most useful ways to think about nutrition for healthspan is this: food is not just fuel. It is information. Every meal sends signals to your cells — signals that influence gene expression, hormonal balance, inflammatory pathways, the gut microbiome, and dozens of other biological processes that collectively determine your rate of biological ageing.

The research on nutrition is messier and more contested than the research on sleep or exercise. But the broad outlines are clear enough to act on. Eat plenty of whole, minimally processed plant foods. Meet your protein needs, especially as you age. Minimise ultra-processed foods. Choose quality fats. Manage your carbohydrate quality. Stay hydrated. Eat socially when you can.

You do not need to be perfect. You do not need to follow a named diet. You do not need to spend a fortune on superfoods. You need to make consistent choices that shift the balance of your dietary pattern in the direction the evidence supports — and then let the compounding effect of those choices work over years and decades.

Food is one of the great pleasures of life. The evidence-based approach to nutrition for healthspan does not require you to surrender that pleasure. It asks you to bring more of it to the table — literally.

Chapter Summary

- The Mediterranean dietary pattern — abundant in vegetables, legumes, whole grains, olive oil, and fish — is consistently associated with a 23 per cent reduction in all-cause mortality across large, well-powered studies.

- Ultra-processed foods are directly associated with 32 adverse health outcomes. The highest UPF consumers have a 15 per cent greater all-cause mortality risk. The mechanisms include gut dysbiosis, inflammation, disrupted appetite signalling, and nutrient displacement.

- Protein intake is the most underrated nutritional issue for ageing adults. Australia's current NHMRC NRVs (2006) set the RDI at 0.75–0.84g/kg/day, but these are under review. The clinical evidence — including ESPEN guidelines and multiple meta-analyses — supports 1.2–1.6g/kg/day for most adults over 50, with higher targets during illness or active resistance training.

- Protein distribution across meals matters: 25–40g of high-quality protein per meal is needed to maximally stimulate muscle protein synthesis in older adults.

- Omega-3 fatty acids (EPA/DHA from oily fish), dietary fibre (25–30g/day), and polyphenols from colourful plant foods all have strong supporting evidence for healthspan.

- Blood glucose management through carbohydrate quality — prioritising low-GI whole food sources over refined carbohydrates and added sugars — is a key nutritional lever for metabolic health.

- Time-restricted eating (12:12 or 10:14 patterns) has a sound biological rationale and early evidence for metabolic benefit, though older adults should ensure adequate protein and total calorie intake within the eating window.

- Supplements worth considering for many Australians include vitamin D, omega-3, magnesium, creatine (for resistance training), and B12 (particularly for those over 60 or on metformin). Test before supplementing where possible.

References

Ahmad, S., Moorthy, M. V., Lee, I. M., Ridker, P. M., Manson, J. E., & Mora, S. (2024). Mediterranean diet adherence and risk of all-cause mortality in women. JAMA Network Open, 7(5), e2414322. https://doi.org/10.1001/jamanetworkopen.2024.14322

Furbatto, M., Lelli, D., Antonelli Incalzi, R., & Pedone, C. (2024). Mediterranean diet in older adults: Cardiovascular outcomes and mortality from observational and interventional studies — a systematic review and meta-analysis. Nutrients, 16(22), 3947.

Lane, M. M., Gamage, E., Du, S., Ashtree, D. N., McGuinness, A. J., Gauci, S., et al. (2024). Ultra-processed food exposure and adverse health outcomes: umbrella review of epidemiological meta-analyses. BMJ, 384, e077310.

Yang, X., et al. (2025). Ultra-processed foods and risk of all-cause mortality: an updated systematic review and dose-response meta-analysis of prospective cohort studies. Systematic Reviews. https://doi.org/10.1186/s13643-025-02800-8

Torres-Collado, L., et al. (2024). A high consumption of ultra-processed foods is associated with higher total mortality in an adult Mediterranean population. Clinical Nutrition, 43, 739–746.

Deutz, N. E. P., et al. (2014). Protein intake and exercise for optimal muscle function with aging: recommendations from the ESPEN Expert Group. Clinical Nutrition, 33(6), 929–936.

Groenendijk, I., de Groot, L. C. P. G. M., Tetens, I., & Grootswagers, P. (2024). Discussion on protein recommendations for supporting muscle and bone health in older adults: a mini review. Frontiers in Nutrition, 11, 1394916.

Ishaq, F., et al. (2025). Role of protein intake in maintaining muscle mass composition among elderly females suffering from sarcopenia. Frontiers in Nutrition. https://doi.org/10.3389/fnut.2025.1547325

Hu, F. B. (2024). Diet strategies for promoting healthy aging and longevity: an epidemiological perspective. Journal of Internal Medicine, 295, 508–531.

Sebastian, S. A., Padda, I., & Johal, G. (2024). Long-term impact of Mediterranean diet on cardiovascular disease prevention: a systematic review and meta-analysis. Current Problems in Cardiology, 49(5), 102509.

Chapter Seven

Stress and the Nervous System

---

*How chronic stress accelerates ageing
— and what you can actually do about
it*

Stress is often dismissed as a soft problem. We talk about it in the break room, mention it apologetically to our GP, and quietly accept it as the unavoidable price of modern life. It is not something we typically think of as a biological process with measurable molecular consequences — as something that shortens our telomeres, accelerates our epigenetic age, promotes cellular senescence, drives inflammation, and meaningfully increases our risk of heart disease, cancer, and dementia.

But that is exactly what chronic stress does. The evidence, accumulated over decades across human cohort studies, animal models, and mechanistic research, is now clear enough to be unambiguous: sustained psychological stress is not merely unpleasant. It is a driver of accelerated biological ageing, operating through multiple overlapping pathways that touch virtually every hallmark of ageing described in Chapter One.

This does not mean that all stress is harmful — far from it. Acute, manageable stress is not only normal but necessary. It sharpens cognitive performance, motivates adaptive responses, and when resolved,

123

leaves the body stronger and more resilient. The problem is not stress per se. The problem is chronic, unresolved stress that keeps the body's alarm systems activated long after the threat has passed.

Understanding how the stress response works biologically — and where it goes wrong — is the foundation for understanding why stress management is a genuine medical priority, not a luxury. And understanding the evidence-based interventions for chronic stress gives you practical tools to address it in your own life.

The Stress Response: Designed for Survival, Not Modernity

The biological stress response is one of evolution's most elegant achievements. When the brain perceives a threat — whether a predator, a social confrontation, a looming deadline, or a frightening news headline — a cascade of physiological changes is triggered within milliseconds. Heart rate and blood pressure rise. Glucose floods the bloodstream. Blood is diverted from digestive organs to muscles. The immune system enters a state of alert. Pain sensitivity drops. Cognitive focus sharpens.

This response is orchestrated by two interlocking systems. The first — fast and immediate — is the sympathetic-adrenal-medullary (SAM) axis, which triggers the release of adrenaline and noradrenaline from the adrenal glands. This is the 'fight or flight' response: it prepares you for immediate physical action within seconds. The second — slightly slower but more sustained — is the hypothalamic-pituitary-adrenal (HPA) axis, which triggers the release of cortisol from the adrenal cortex. Cortisol is the principal stress hormone: it mobilises energy, modulates immune responses, and helps sustain the stress response over minutes to hours.

Both systems evolved in an environment where most threats were acute: physical danger that was either overcome or fled from, followed by a period of recovery. The stress response resolved. Cortisol levels returned to baseline. The nervous system shifted back to its parasympathetic 'rest and digest' mode.

Modern stressors — financial pressure, workplace demands, relationship conflict, health anxiety, social comparison, information overload — are rarely resolved so cleanly. They are persistent, diffuse, often uncontrollable, and many operate in the background continuously. The result is a nervous system that never fully returns to baseline: a state of chronic low-level activation that, over months and years, generates a significant biological cost.

"The human stress response evolved to manage acute physical threats. It was not designed for the relentless, unresolvable pressures of modern life."

How Chronic Stress Accelerates Biological Ageing

A 2024 review published in Frontiers in Ageing synthesised the mechanistic evidence linking chronic psychological stress to each of the major hallmarks of ageing. The conclusion was clear: chronic stress activates and accelerates virtually every known biological pathway of ageing, simultaneously and in ways that reinforce each other (Wang et al., 2024).

Telomere Attrition

The link between chronic stress and accelerated telomere shortening is one of the most replicated findings in psychoneuroimmunology. Cortisol suppresses telomerase — the enzyme responsible for maintaining and repairing telomere length — while simultaneously increasing oxidative stress and inflammation, both of which damage telomeric DNA directly. People in chronically stressful circumstances — caregivers, those experiencing adversity, those in high-demand low-control occupations — consistently show shorter telomeres than age-matched controls (Souza-Talarico et al., 2024).

The seminal work of Nobel laureate Elizabeth Blackburn and her colleague Elissa Epel demonstrated that caregivers of chronically ill children had significantly shorter telomeres than non-caregivers, and that the degree of shortening correlated with the perceived level of stress rather than the objective caregiving burden. This was a landmark finding: it was not the circumstances themselves but the subjective experience of those circumstances that drove the biological impact.

Epigenetic Acceleration

Chronic stress produces measurable epigenetic age acceleration — a direct demonstration, using methylation clocks of the kind discussed in Chapter Two, that sustained stress biologically ages people faster. Studies of individuals exposed to early life adversity, occupational burnout, and prolonged caregiving consistently show epigenetic ages years ahead of their chronological ages. Cortisol appears to directly influence DNA methylation patterns at specific sites involved in immune regulation, inflammatory signalling, and metabolic control.

Inflammageing

One of the most important downstream effects of chronic HPA and SAM axis activation is a persistent shift towards a pro-inflammatory state. Cortisol, in the short term, is anti-inflammatory. But chronic cortisol exposure leads to cortisol resistance in immune cells — they stop responding appropriately to cortisol's suppressive signals — and inflammatory cytokines including IL-6, TNF-alpha, and CRP become chronically elevated. This is one of the principal mechanisms through which chronic stress drives the inflammageing discussed in Chapter One, and through which it increases risk of cardiovascular disease, metabolic dysfunction, depression, and cancer.

Mitochondrial Dysfunction

Stress hormones — particularly glucocorticoids and catecholamines — directly impair mitochondrial function, reducing energy production efficiency and increasing the generation of reactive oxygen species (ROS). This mitochondrial stress is amplified by the fact that chronically stressed individuals often sleep poorly, exercise less, and eat in ways that further compromise mitochondrial health — creating a compounding negative loop.

Cellular Senescence

Chronic oxidative stress, DNA damage, and inflammatory signalling — all promoted by chronic HPA activation — accelerate the rate at which cells enter senescence. Senescent cells, as discussed in Chapter One, do not die — they persist in tissue, secreting inflammatory molecules that further drive systemic inflammation and neighbouring cell dysfunction. Elevated allostatic load — the cumulative biological wear and tear of chronic stress — is now consistently associated with higher burdens of senescent cells.

Allostatic Load: Measuring the Cost of Chronic Stress

The concept of allostatic load — originally proposed by neuroscientist Bruce McEwen in the 1990s — provides one of the most clinically useful frameworks for understanding how chronic stress translates into disease. Allostasis is the process by which the body adapts to stress by changing its physiological set points. Allostatic load is the cumulative cost of those adaptations over time: the biological wear and tear that accumulates when stress systems are repeatedly or chronically activated.

Allostatic load is measurable. It is assessed by combining biomarkers across multiple physiological systems — cardiovascular (blood pressure, resting heart rate), metabolic (fasting glucose, HbA1c, waist-to-hip ratio), inflammatory (CRP, IL-6), and neuroendocrine (cortisol, DHEA) — to create a composite score that reflects the cumulative biological burden of chronic stress. Higher allostatic load scores are associated with accelerated biological ageing, greater all-cause mortality, cardiovascular disease, cognitive decline, and a wide range of mental health disorders.

Importantly, allostatic load is modifiable. Interventions that reduce chronic stress — exercise, sleep, mindfulness, social connection, psychological therapy, and lifestyle change — produce measurable reductions in allostatic load biomarkers. This makes allostatic load not just a diagnostic concept but a target for intervention.

In a clinical context, asking your GP for a basic panel that includes blood pressure, fasting glucose, HbA1c, waist circumference, and CRP gives you a reasonable proxy for your allostatic load — and provides actionable targets for improvement.

7 hallmarks of ageing that chronic stress directly activates or accelerates

~45% of Australians reported significant stress in the past year (APS Stress and Wellbeing Survey)

23% shorter telomeres in high-stress caregivers compared to low-stress controls in landmark studies

8 weeks duration of MBSR programs in most well-powered studies, producing measurable reductions in cortisol and inflammatory markers

The Autonomic Nervous System: Your Internal Stress Regulator

Understanding how to practically manage stress requires understanding one more piece of biology: the autonomic nervous system (ANS). The ANS operates largely below conscious awareness, regulating heart rate, breathing, digestion, immune activity, and dozens of other involuntary functions. It has two major branches that operate in dynamic balance.

The sympathetic nervous system (SNS) — the 'fight or flight' system — accelerates heart rate, increases blood pressure, diverts blood to muscles, inhibits digestion, and mobilises energy. It is activated by perceived threat or demand.

The parasympathetic nervous system (PNS) — the 'rest and digest' or 'rest and repair' system — does the opposite: it slows heart rate, lowers blood pressure, promotes digestion and immune surveillance, and supports cellular repair. It is the biological state of recovery.

The balance between these two systems is reflected in a measure called heart rate variability (HRV) — the variation in the time interval between successive heartbeats. Higher HRV indicates greater parasympathetic dominance, better autonomic flexibility, and greater stress resilience. Lower HRV — more common in chronically stressed, unfit, or ageing individuals — indicates sympathetic dominance and reduced capacity for recovery.

HRV is now easily measurable through consumer wearables including the Apple Watch, Garmin, Whoop, and Oura Ring, and has become one of the most widely used practical markers of stress and recovery status. A sustained decline in your baseline HRV is one of the earliest and most sensitive indicators that your nervous system is carrying more stress than it can effectively process.

The therapeutic implication is direct: interventions that increase parasympathetic tone — slow diaphragmatic breathing, mindfulness, aerobic exercise, adequate sleep, time in nature — are not just relaxation techniques. They are producing measurable changes in autonomic balance that have downstream effects on immune function, inflammatory markers, cardiovascular health, and biological ageing.

Evidence-Based Stress Management: What Actually Works

The stress management space is unfortunately crowded with low-quality interventions and high-quality marketing. The following summary focuses specifically on interventions with meaningful evidence from well-designed clinical trials and systematic reviews.

Mindfulness-Based Stress Reduction (MBSR)

Of all the psychological stress management interventions studied, Mindfulness-Based Stress Reduction — an eight-week structured programme developed by Jon Kabat-Zinn at the University of Massachusetts — has the most robust evidence base. A 2024 systematic review of mindfulness-based interventions and the HPA axis confirmed that MBSR produces significant reductions in cortisol, reductions in sympathetic nervous system activity, and improvements in autonomic balance. An 89-study meta-analysis of mind-body interventions published in 2025 confirmed that MBSR and comparable programmes reduced pro-inflammatory cytokines including IL-6 and TNF-alpha, and increased markers of immune competence.

The neurobiological evidence is also compelling. Systematic reviews published in 2024 found that mindfulness practice induces measurable neuroplasticity: increased cortical thickness in areas associated with emotional regulation, reduced amygdala reactivity to stress, and improved connectivity between the prefrontal cortex (rational control) and limbic system (emotional reactivity). These are not subtle or transient effects — they represent structural changes in the brain that persist beyond the training period.

MBSR is available in Australia through psychologists, mindfulness-based cognitive therapy (MBCT) programmes, and increasingly through online platforms. The Smiling Mind app, developed in Australia, provides a free, accessible introduction to mindfulness practice and is backed by outcome research in Australian populations. For those with significant anxiety or trauma, engaging a trained psychologist for MBCT or MBSR is strongly recommended over solo app-based practice.

Exercise

Exercise is not just a physical health intervention — it is one of the most powerful nervous system regulators available. Aerobic exercise increases parasympathetic tone, improves HRV, reduces basal cortisol, promotes the release of BDNF (which supports brain resilience), and reduces inflammatory markers. A single bout of moderate-intensity aerobic exercise produces an immediate and measurable reduction in psychological stress and anxiety. Over time, regular aerobic training produces sustained improvements in HRV and stress resilience that persist even under acute stress conditions.

The relationship between exercise and stress management is bidirectional: exercise reduces the physiological impact of stress, and it also builds the neurobiological resilience that makes future stressors less destabilising. People who exercise regularly consistently report lower perceived stress and higher psychological wellbeing, and the mechanistic evidence supports this as a genuine biological effect rather than simply a distraction or mood boost.

Controlled Breathing

Deliberate regulation of the breath is one of the fastest and most accessible ways to shift the autonomic nervous system from sympathetic to parasympathetic dominance. The vagus nerve — the principal nerve of the parasympathetic system — is activated by slow, diaphragmatic breathing, producing immediate reductions in heart rate, blood pressure, and cortisol release.

The most well-studied breathing protocol is slow breathing at approximately five to six breath cycles per minute — roughly five seconds in and five seconds out — which produces what researchers call 'resonance frequency breathing', maximising the coherence and amplitude of HRV. Even five to ten minutes of this practice produces measurable and clinically significant changes in autonomic balance. Longer-term practice (eight or more weeks of daily slow breathing) produces lasting improvements in basal HRV.

Box breathing (four seconds in, four seconds hold, four seconds out, four seconds hold) and the 4-7-8 breathing technique are also effective and accessible. These are not elaborate protocols — they are simple, evidence-based tools that can be deployed in any stressful moment, requiring no equipment and no formal training.

Nature Exposure and Social Connection

Two factors with growing evidence bases deserve specific mention: time in natural environments and quality social connection. Research consistently shows that exposure to natural settings — forests, coastlines, parks, gardens — reduces cortisol, lowers blood pressure, improves HRV, and reduces inflammatory markers. A meta-analysis of 'green space' interventions found significant and consistent reductions in salivary cortisol. Given Australia's extraordinary natural environment, this is a particularly accessible and underused intervention.

Social connection is covered in depth in Chapter Eight, but its relationship to the stress response deserves mention here. Chronic social isolation activates the HPA and SAM axes in ways that are biologically analogous to other stressors, producing elevated cortisol, increased inflammation, and accelerated biological ageing. Conversely, strong social connection buffers the stress response — the presence of trusted others reduces the cortisol and cardiovascular response to acute stressors. Loneliness is a physiological stressor, and addressing it is a legitimate and important stress management strategy.

Psychological Therapy

For people whose stress is rooted in identifiable psychological patterns — rumination, perfectionism, difficulty with boundaries, trauma responses, anxiety disorders — professional psychological support is not a last resort. It is often the most targeted and lasting intervention available. Cognitive Behavioural Therapy (CBT), Acceptance and Commitment Therapy (ACT), and psychodynamic therapies all have evidence bases for reducing chronic stress and its physiological consequences. In Australia, GP Mental Health Treatment Plans provide partial Medicare rebates for up to ten psychology sessions per year, making this meaningfully more accessible than it might otherwise be.

A Practical Stress Management Framework

No single intervention addresses all dimensions of chronic stress. The most effective approach combines multiple evidence-based strategies across different time frames — immediate tools for acute stress moments, regular practices that build ongoing resilience, and structural changes that reduce the sources of chronic stress themselves.

Time Frame	Strategy	Practical Application
Immediate (minutes)	Slow breathing / box breathing	5–10 min of slow diaphragmatic breathing (5–6 breaths/min). Use in any acute stress moment.

Time Frame	Strategy	Practical Application
Daily (10–20 min)	Mindfulness practice	Guided meditation app (Smiling Mind, Insight Timer) or formal MBSR programme. Morning practice is most consistent.
Daily	Physical activity	Even a 20–30 min walk produces measurable stress-reduction. Exercise is a nervous system regulator, not just physical training.
Daily	Nature time	Time outdoors in green or blue spaces. Even urban parks reduce cortisol measurably. Combine with walking if possible.
Daily	Sleep protection	Sleep is when the HPA axis resets. Chronic poor sleep perpetuates stress physiology. Protecting sleep quality is stress management.
Weekly	Social connection	Prioritise meaningful in-person connection. Quality matters more than quantity. Loneliness is a physiological stressor.

Time Frame	Strategy	Practical Application
Ongoing	HRV monitoring	Wearable devices provide real-time feedback on nervous system recovery. Use as an early warning system, not a source of new anxiety.
As needed	Psychological therapy	CBT, ACT, or MBCT with a registered psychologist via GP Mental Health Treatment Plan. Partial Medicare rebate, up to 10 sessions/year.
Structural	Source reduction	Identify and address chronic stressors where possible: unsustainable workloads, relationship difficulties, financial pressures. Coping is necessary; elimination is better.

Stress in the Australian Context

Australian data consistently shows that stress is a significant and under addressed public health issue. The Australian Psychological Society's annual Stress and Wellbeing surveys have repeatedly found that nearly half of Australians report significant stress in the preceding year, with work, finances, and personal health among the most common sources. The consequences are visible in the rates of anxiety and depression, cardiovascular disease, and metabolic dysfunction that characterise the Australian disease burden.

There is a cultural dimension worth acknowledging. The Australian tendency to minimise emotional difficulty — the 'she'll be right' ethos — is both a genuine strength in some contexts and a barrier to help-seeking in others. Men in particular are significantly less likely than women to seek professional support for stress or psychological distress, despite comparable rates of chronic stress exposure. The under-utilisation of GP Mental Health Treatment Plans and psychological services in Australia, particularly among working-age men, represents a significant gap between the availability of effective intervention and its uptake.

The good news is that not all stress management requires professional help or significant time investment. The evidence-based tools described in this chapter — controlled breathing, regular exercise, mindfulness, time outdoors, and deliberate investment in social connection — are accessible to virtually every Australian, in every postcode, at minimal cost. They do not require a formal diagnosis or a practitioner referral. They require only the recognition that managing stress is a genuine medical priority, not an indulgence.

Stress Is Not Inevitable — It Is Manageable

I want to be direct about something that patients sometimes find difficult to hear: the way you manage stress is not a minor lifestyle detail. It is a determinant of how quickly your cells age, how well your immune system functions, and how long you spend in good health.

The research is clear. Chronic unmanaged stress shortens telomeres, accelerates epigenetic ageing, promotes inflammation, impairs mitochondrial function, and increases the risk of virtually every major age-related disease. It is not possible to optimise your healthspan while running a chronically activated stress response.

But the research is equally clear on something else: the stress response is modifiable. The nervous system is plastic. The HPA axis can recalibrate. Biological age acceleration driven by chronic stress can, with appropriate intervention, be slowed and partially reversed. The tools exist. The evidence supports them. The question is whether you are prepared to treat managing your nervous system as seriously as you treat managing your blood pressure or your cholesterol.

You should. The biological stakes are the same.

Chapter Summary

- Chronic psychological stress is a direct driver of accelerated biological ageing, activating and accelerating seven of the twelve hallmarks of ageing simultaneously.

- The HPA axis (cortisol) and SAM axis (adrenaline/noradrenaline) are the two principal stress response systems. Acute stress is adaptive; chronic activation without recovery is biologically costly.

- Key mechanisms through which chronic stress ages the body include: telomere attrition (cortisol suppresses telomerase), epigenetic acceleration, chronic inflammation (inflammageing), mitochondrial dysfunction, and accelerated cellular senescence.

- Allostatic load is the cumulative biological cost of chronic stress, measurable through biomarkers across cardiovascular, metabolic, neuroendocrine, and inflammatory systems. It is modifiable through lifestyle and psychological intervention.

- Heart rate variability (HRV) is a practical, accessible marker of autonomic balance and stress resilience. Consumer wearables make daily HRV monitoring feasible and informative.

- The most evidence-based stress management interventions are: MBSR/mindfulness (reduces cortisol, improves brain structure), exercise (improves HRV and reduces inflammatory markers), slow controlled breathing (immediate parasympathetic activation), nature exposure (reduces cortisol), social connection (buffers the stress response), and psychological therapy (CBT, ACT, MBCT).

- In Australia, GP Mental Health Treatment Plans provide partial Medicare rebates for up to ten psychology sessions per year — a significantly underutilised pathway.

- Treating stress management as a medical priority — not a lifestyle indulgence — is one of the most important reframes for anyone serious about their long-term healthspan.

References

Wang, Y., et al. (2024). Molecular pathways linking chronic psychological stress to accelerated aging: mechanisms and interventions. Frontiers in Aging. https://doi.org/10.3389/fragi.2026.1743142

Souza-Talarico, J. N., et al. (2024). Exploring the interplay of psychological and biological components of stress response and telomere length in the transition from middle age to late adulthood: A systematic review. Stress and Health, 40(4), e3389.

Bartolo, A., et al. (2023). The impact of life stress on hallmarks of aging and accelerated senescence: connections in sickness and in health. Neuroscience & Biobehavioral Reviews, 153, 105359. https://pmc.ncbi.nlm.nih.gov/articles/PMC10592082/

Epel, E. S., Blackburn, E. H., Lin, J., et al. (2004). Accelerated telomere shortening in response to life stress. Proceedings of the National Academy of Sciences, 101(49), 17312–17315.

Sáez, H., et al. (2024). Mindfulness-based interventions and the hypothalamic–pituitary–adrenal axis: A systematic review. Nutrients, 16(6), 115. https://pmc.ncbi.nlm.nih.gov/articles/PMC11587421/

Li, S., et al. (2025). Effects of mind–body interventions on immune and neuroendocrine functions: a systematic review and meta-analysis of randomized controlled trials. Healthcare, 13(8), 952.

Diez, I., et al. (2024). Neurobiological changes induced by mindfulness and meditation: a systematic review. Brain Sciences, 14(11). https://pmc.ncbi.nlm.nih.gov/articles/PMC11591838/

Kiecolt-Glaser, J. K., et al. (2020). Contemplative practices and allostatic load: A synthesis of research on mindfulness-based interventions and biomarkers of stress. Psychosomatic Medicine, 82(5), 447–460.

McEwen, B. S. (2007). Physiology and neurobiology of stress and adaptation: central role of the brain. Physiological Reviews, 87(3), 873–904.

Australian Psychological Society. (2023). Stress and Wellbeing in Australia Survey 2023. APS. https://psychology.org.au

Chapter Eight

Connection and Purpose

The underrated pillars of a long, well life — and why belonging and meaning are not soft extras

Of all the factors that determine how long and how well we live, two are consistently underestimated — not because the evidence for them is weak, but because they do not fit neatly into the biomedical model of health that dominates both clinical practice and popular health culture. We are very good at talking about diet, exercise, and sleep. We are considerably less comfortable acknowledging that the quality of our relationships and the presence of meaning in our lives are, by every measurable biological standard, just as important.

The research on this is unambiguous. Strong social connection is one of the most powerful predictors of longevity ever identified. The absence of it — loneliness and social isolation — is associated with mortality risk comparable to smoking fifteen cigarettes a day. A sense of purpose in life predicts survival, cognitive preservation, and disease resistance in ways that no supplement or medication comes close to matching.

These are not soft findings. They are replicated across large cohort studies, meta-analyses of millions of people, and mechanistic research that reveals clear biological pathways through which connection and purpose influence the body at the cellular level. If social relationships and life purpose were drugs, they would be prescribed immediately and universally. Because they are not drugs, they tend to get mentioned briefly in health consultations and then left for the individual to figure out.

This chapter is about taking that seriously.

The Mortality Evidence: Social Connection Saves Lives

In 2010, Julianne Holt-Lunstad and colleagues at Brigham Young University published what has become one of the most cited studies in social epidemiology: a meta-analysis of 148 studies examining the protective effect of social connection on survival, with data from over 300,000 participants. The finding was striking: strong social relationships increased the odds of survival by 50 per cent, across a diverse range of populations, age groups, and health conditions (Holt-Lunstad et al., 2010).

A 2015 follow-up meta-analysis examined the flip side — the mortality risk associated with loneliness, social isolation, and living alone. Across 70 studies with over 3.4 million participants, social isolation was associated with a 29 per cent increase in mortality risk, loneliness with a 26 per cent increase, and living alone with a 32 per cent increase. These effects were independent of physical health status, age, and other confounders — and they were comparable in magnitude to well-established risk factors like smoking and obesity (Holt-Lunstad et al., 2015).

A comprehensive 2024 review published in World Psychiatry by Holt-Lunstad synthesised two decades of evidence and concluded that social connection remains one of the strongest independent predictors of both mental and physical health outcomes, with particularly robust evidence on mortality. The review noted that societal trends across multiple indicators show increasing rates of social disconnection — and that the biological and health consequences of this trend are substantial and growing.

"Strong social relationships increase the odds of survival by 50%. Loneliness is associated with a 26% increase in mortality risk — comparable to smoking 15 cigarettes a day." — Holt-Lunstad, 2010, 2015

The 2025 meta-analysis published in the European Archives of Psychiatry and Clinical Neuroscience, examining 86 studies of older adults specifically, confirmed that loneliness, social isolation, and living alone are all significant independent risk factors for all-cause and cause-specific mortality in later life. The relationship held across countries, genders, and health conditions.

These findings prompted action at the highest levels. In 2023, the US Surgeon General issued a formal Advisory declaring an 'epidemic of loneliness and isolation', calling it a fundamental public health threat. In January 2024, governments of six countries — including the United States, Japan, Sweden, and others — issued a joint statement highlighting social connection as a critical public health priority. Australia has not yet appointed a Minister for Loneliness as the UK and Japan have, but the AIHW has acknowledged social isolation and loneliness as a recognised public health concern in its welfare reporting.

Why Social Connection Affects Biology: The Mechanisms

The question of how human relationships produce measurable effects on survival, cardiovascular disease, cancer risk, and dementia is now well understood at a mechanistic level. The human need for social connection is not a cultural preference or a psychological luxury — it is wired into our neurobiology.

The Stress Buffering Effect

As discussed in Chapter Seven, chronic HPA axis activation — sustained cortisol release — drives inflammation, telomere attrition, epigenetic ageing, and accelerated disease across virtually every organ system. Social connection directly moderates this response. The presence of trusted others reduces cortisol output in response to acute stressors, dampens the inflammatory response, and promotes parasympathetic recovery. Research consistently shows that the same objective stressor produces significantly different physiological responses in people who are socially connected compared to those who are isolated. Connection is a biological buffer against the ageing effects of stress.

Inflammation and Immune Function

Chronic loneliness produces a distinct and measurable biological signature. People experiencing persistent loneliness show elevated levels of pro-inflammatory cytokines — particularly IL-6, IL-1 beta, and CRP — and dysregulated immune responses. John Cacioppo's pioneering research demonstrated that lonely individuals show upregulation of genes associated with inflammation and downregulation of genes associated with antiviral responses and antibody production. This 'loneliness transcriptome' — a characteristic pattern of gene expression — helps explain why lonely people are not only more susceptible to infection but also more vulnerable to the inflammatory diseases of ageing.

The Nervous System

Social isolation activates the same neural threat-detection circuits that respond to physical danger, producing sustained sympathetic nervous system arousal, elevated cortisol, and the cascade of physiological consequences that follow. Conversely, positive social connection activates the parasympathetic nervous system, promotes oxytocin release, and creates the conditions for biological recovery and repair. In the language of the previous chapter: belonging is a parasympathetic experience. Isolation is a sympathetic one. The cumulative biological cost of prolonged social isolation is, in effect, chronic stress — with all the accelerated ageing that entails.

Behavioural Pathways

Social connection also influences health through behavioural mechanisms. People with strong social networks exercise more, eat better, sleep more consistently, seek medical help more readily, and are more likely to adhere to treatment. They have more accountability, more incentive, and more practical support. The biological mechanisms and the behavioural mechanisms are not competing explanations — they operate simultaneously, which is part of why the mortality effect of social connection is so large.

The Australian Picture: Loneliness as a Public Health Issue

Loneliness and social isolation are not abstract global trends — they are pressing realities in the Australian community. The AIHW reports that approximately 16 per cent of older Australians aged over 65 experience loneliness, with rates rising to 19 per cent in those aged 75 and over. Prior to the COVID-19 pandemic, approximately one in five older Australians were socially isolated. The pandemic significantly worsened both measures — and the recovery has been incomplete.

Importantly, loneliness is not exclusively a problem of older adults. AIHW data from Australia's Welfare 2023 showed that people aged 18 to 24 reported the highest levels of loneliness throughout the pandemic period, and the frequency of social contact has been declining across all age groups for decades. Social media use has increased, but its substitution for the quality of in-person connection is imperfect at best — and for many, counterproductive.

The total cost of loneliness to the Australian economy was estimated at approximately $2.7 billion — around $1,565 per person who becomes or remains lonely — largely driven by increased health service use, including general practice and hospital visits. Lonely older Australians visit GPs and emergency departments more frequently, partially to meet needs for human contact that the healthcare system is poorly designed to address.

A perspective published in the Medical Journal of Australia in 2024 highlighted the need for interventions tailored to the diverse Australian population — including culturally and linguistically diverse communities, LGBTQIA+, older people, Indigenous Australians, and those in rural and remote areas — recognising that loneliness and social isolation manifest differently and require different solutions across these groups.

50% increase in survival odds associated with strong social relationships (Holt-Lunstad et al., 2010)

~1 in 5 older Australians experience social isolation; rates are higher in aged care and rural areas (AIHW)

50% higher risk of all-cause mortality associated with lacking a sense of ikigai in the Ohsaki Study (43,391 participants)

36% lower risk of dementia in older adults with ikigai vs those without, in a large Japanese longitudinal study

Purpose in Life: The Biology of Meaning

Alongside connection, the evidence for purpose in life as a determinant of health and longevity has grown substantially. The concept is perhaps best embodied by the Japanese idea of ikigai — typically translated as 'that which makes life worth living' — a sense that your days have meaning, that there is something worth getting up for, that your presence in the world matters.

The research on purpose and longevity is now extensive. The Ohsaki Study — a prospective cohort of over 43,000 Japanese adults — found that those who did not have a sense of ikigai had a 50 per cent higher risk of all-cause mortality over seven years, with the excess risk driven primarily by cardiovascular disease and external causes (Tanno et al., 2009). A landmark study published in JAMA Network Open in 2019 followed 6,985 US adults over 50 and found that a strong sense of purpose was associated with significantly reduced all-cause and cardiovascular mortality over four years (Alimujiang et al., 2019).

A longitudinal study published in 2022 using data from over 6,000 Japanese older adults found that those with ikigai had a 31 per cent lower risk of developing functional disability and a 36 per cent lower risk of developing dementia over three years, independent of health status, socioeconomic factors, and baseline function (Okuzono et al., 2022). Research published in 2025 in ScienceDirect found that ikigai was associated with frailty prevention specifically in women, with the biological mediating mechanism involving reduced inflammatory burden — a finding that connects purpose directly to the inflammageing discussed in Chapter One.

How does purpose in life produce these biological effects? Several mechanisms are now established. People with strong purpose show reduced HPA axis reactivity to stress — their cortisol responses to acute stressors are more regulated, and their recovery is faster. They show lower basal levels of inflammatory markers including IL-6 and CRP. They engage more consistently in health-promoting behaviours. And emerging research suggests they show reduced epigenetic ageing — purpose correlates with younger biological ages on methylation clocks, suggesting a genuine cellular anti-ageing effect of meaning.

The Blue Zones Perspective

The Blue Zones — the five regions of the world identified by National Geographic researcher Dan Buettner where people live measurably longer, healthier lives — offer a complementary lens on purpose and connection. These regions (Sardinia in Italy, Okinawa in Japan, the Nicoya Peninsula in Costa Rica, Ikaria in Greece, and Loma Linda in California) share a number of consistent features, not all of which are dietary. Among the most consistent: strong social bonds and community belonging, regular engagement with a multigenerational community, a clear sense of life purpose, and deep integration of meaningful activity throughout old age.

In Okinawa, the concept of ikigai is central to how elders understand their daily life. In Sardinia, the strong tradition of community celebration and multigenerational household ensures that old people remain valued, seen, and socially embedded. In all five zones, social isolation is structurally rare — not because people are specially virtuous, but because the environment makes connection easy and expected.

The lesson from the Blue Zones is not that we should replicate Sardinian culture or adopt Okinawan diet wholesale. It is that the physical and social environments we live in either support or undermine connection and purpose — and that individual behaviour change, while important, operates within those environmental constraints. The 1st World Longevity Summit, held in Kyotango Japan in 2025, formally identified ikigai and social bonds as two of four pillars of healthy longevity alongside dietary fibre and physical activity.

Practical Strategies: Building Connection and Cultivating Purpose

The evidence is clear that connection and purpose are not fixed traits — they are cultivatable, and their cultivation produces measurable biological and health benefits. The following strategies are grounded in both the research evidence and practical clinical experience.

On Building Connection

- Prioritise quality over quantity. The research consistently shows that the depth and perceived quality of social relationships matters more than their number. A few close, trusting relationships contribute more to health than a large but superficial social network.

- Invest in existing relationships deliberately. Relationships require maintenance — time, attention, and reciprocity. Scheduling regular contact with people who matter to you is not over-engineering friendship; it is recognising that important things rarely happen without intention.

- Build connection through shared activity. The most durable social bonds tend to form around shared purpose or activity — sport, volunteering, community organisations, creative pursuits, religious or spiritual communities. Activity-based connection is particularly powerful because it also addresses purpose simultaneously.

- Reduce barriers to social engagement. Common barriers — busyness, transport, financial cost, physical mobility, social anxiety — deserve direct problem-solving. If social anxiety is a significant barrier, a brief course of CBT with a psychologist can produce lasting improvement. This is a legitimate use of a GP Mental Health Treatment Plan.

- Be aware of the quality of digital connection. Online contact is not equivalent to in-person interaction for many of the biological mechanisms discussed above — oxytocin release, parasympathetic activation, and stress buffering are particularly dependent on physical presence. Use digital connection as a supplement to in-person contact, not a replacement for it.

- Transition points are high risk. Retirement, bereavement, relocation, health change, and the departure of adult children are all life transitions that commonly erode social connection. Proactively building new social infrastructure during these transitions — rather than waiting to feel lonely — is one of the most important social health strategies available.

On Cultivating Purpose

- Take the question seriously. 'What gives my life meaning?' is not a question for philosophers or people in crisis. It is a health question with measurable biological consequences. Many people never ask it explicitly. It is worth asking — and sitting with.

- Distinguish purpose from goals. Goals are specific, time-bound, and can be completed. Purpose is directional, ongoing, and expands rather than concludes. A goal is 'I want to get fit'. A purpose is 'I want to be someone who shows up physically and mentally for the people I love.' The shift in framing is meaningful.

- Look for multiple sources. People who rely on a single source of purpose — work, for example — are particularly vulnerable when that source disappears at retirement. Cultivating purpose across multiple domains (relationships, creative work, community contribution, spiritual practice, personal growth) creates resilience.

- Contribution matters. Research consistently shows that prosocial behaviour — volunteering, mentoring, helping others — is among the most reliable ways to access a sense of purpose, and produces measurable health benefits including reduced inflammatory markers and improved longevity. The AIHW specifically identifies volunteering as a safeguard against loneliness and social isolation.

- Physical engagement with meaningful activity matters as much as the activity itself. Meaning that is lived and embodied — turning up to the community garden, playing in the band, sitting with a friend who is unwell — produces different biology than meaning that is purely abstract. Get out of your head and into action.

When Loneliness Is Already Established: What Helps

For many Australians — particularly those over 65, those who have recently retired or been bereaved, and those in regional or remote areas — loneliness is not a future risk but a present reality. The evidence on what interventions actually reduce loneliness in older adults is growing, though the evidence base is less mature than for individual-level health interventions.

What the current evidence supports: group-based activities centred on a shared interest or activity are consistently more effective than one-to-one befriending or information provision alone. Educational interventions that build social skills or address maladaptive thought patterns around social connection (consistent with cognitive-behavioural approaches) show good outcomes. Volunteering and reciprocal support — where the person experiencing loneliness also contributes to others — appears particularly effective, possibly because it addresses purpose and connection simultaneously.

In Australia, several evidence-informed pathways exist. GPs can refer older adults to social prescribing through Primary Health Networks (PHNs), which connect people to community activities, volunteer programmes, and group-based services suited to their interests and circumstances. Programs such as Ending Loneliness Together — Australia's national alliance on loneliness — provide resources and program directories for individuals and service providers. The federal government's Aged Care Volunteer Visitors Scheme provides companionship visits to older people who are at risk of isolation. For those with social anxiety that is a barrier to connection, CBT through a GP Mental Health Treatment Plan offers an effective pathway.

For younger Australians experiencing loneliness, the picture is somewhat different — and emerging evidence suggests that loneliness in young adulthood can set trajectories that persist into later life if not addressed. University counselling services, youth mental health organisations such as Headspace and Beyond Blue, and active participation in sport, community organisations, and interest groups all provide entry points.

Belonging and Meaning: The Invisible Pillars

Looking across the five foundations covered in Part Two of this book — sleep, movement, nutrition, stress management, and now connection and purpose — a theme emerges. The interventions with the most robust evidence for extending healthspan are not exotic, expensive, or technologically complex. They are the conditions of a well-lived human life: rest, movement, nourishment, equanimity, belonging, and meaning.

Modern health culture tends to overlook the last two, perhaps because they are harder to quantify or sell. But the biology is clear. Loneliness kills with approximately the same efficiency as a serious physical risk factor. A sense of purpose protects the brain, the heart, and the immune system in ways that money cannot directly buy. The people who age best — in every Blue Zone, in every long-term cohort study — are not the ones with the most perfect diets or the most advanced supplement protocols. They are the ones who feel known, valued, and engaged with something larger than themselves.

Building that is the work of a lifetime. And it is work worth doing.

Chapter Summary

- Strong social connection increases odds of survival by 50%. Loneliness and social isolation carry a 26–32% increase in mortality risk — comparable in magnitude to smoking. This evidence is drawn from meta-analyses of millions of participants.

- The biological mechanisms are now well established: social connection buffers the HPA axis stress response, reduces chronic inflammation, supports immune function, and promotes parasympathetic recovery. Loneliness produces a measurable pro-inflammatory gene expression signature.

- Approximately one in five older Australians is socially isolated, and 16% experience loneliness. Rates are higher in aged care facilities (35–61%), rural and remote areas, and following major life transitions. Social contact frequency has been declining across all age groups in Australia for decades.

- Purpose in life — the Japanese concept of ikigai — is a similarly powerful predictor of healthspan. Those lacking a sense of ikigai have a 50% higher all-cause mortality risk, 31% higher risk of functional disability, and 36% higher risk of dementia in large prospective studies.

- The biology of purpose includes reduced HPA reactivity, lower basal inflammation, more consistent engagement in health-promoting behaviours, and emerging evidence for reduced epigenetic ageing.

- Blue Zones — the world's longest-lived communities — consistently feature strong social bonds, multigenerational community, and clear life purpose as structural features, not individual achievements.

- Evidence-based strategies for connection include: prioritising quality over quantity, investing deliberately in existing relationships, building connection through shared activity, addressing social anxiety through CBT, and proactively managing social connection during life transitions.

- Volunteering and prosocial behaviour are among the most reliable ways to cultivate purpose — and produce measurable health benefits including reduced inflammation and improved longevity. The AIHW specifically identifies volunteering as a safeguard against loneliness.

References

Holt-Lunstad, J., Smith, T. B., & Layton, J. B. (2010). Social relationships and mortality risk: A meta-analytic review. PLoS Medicine, 7(7), e1000316.

Holt-Lunstad, J., Smith, T. B., Baker, M., Harris, T., & Stephenson, D. (2015). Loneliness and social isolation as risk factors for mortality: A meta-analytic review. Perspectives on Psychological Science, 10(2), 227–237.

Holt-Lunstad, J. (2024). Social connection as a critical factor for mental and physical health: evidence, trends, challenges, and future implications. World Psychiatry, 23(3), 312–332. https://doi.org/10.1002/wps.21224

Tanno, K., et al. (2009). Sense of life worth living (ikigai) and mortality in Japan: Ohsaki Study. Psychosomatic Medicine, 71(7), 709–714.

Alimujiang, A., et al. (2019). Association between life purpose and mortality among US adults older than 50 years. JAMA Network Open, 2(5), e194270.

Okuzono, S. S., et al. (2022). Ikigai and subsequent health and wellbeing among Japanese older adults: Longitudinal outcome-wide analysis. The Lancet Regional Health – Western Pacific, 21, 100391.

Son, B.-K., et al. (2025). Ikigai is associated with lower incidence of frailty during a 5-year follow-up in older women: The possible role of interleukin-6. Experimental Gerontology. https://doi.org/10.1016/j.exger.2025.112740

Australian Institute of Health and Welfare (AIHW). (2023). Australia's welfare 2023: data insights — social isolation, loneliness and wellbeing. AIHW, Australian Government.

Engel, L., & Mihalopoulos, C. (2024). The loneliness epidemic: A holistic view of its health and economic implications in older age. The Medical Journal of Australia, 221(6), 290–292.

Naito, Y., et al. (2025). Towards global healthy longevity: report from the 1st World Longevity Summit in Kyotango, Japan. npj Aging. https://doi.org/10.1038/s41514-025-00279-0

Chapter Nine

Hormones and Healthspan

*How the hormonal changes of ageing
affect your body — and when
intervention makes sense*

Few areas of medicine generate as much confusion, controversy, and outright misinformation as the intersection of hormones, ageing, and health. On one side, you have practitioners who treat virtually every symptom in middle-aged patients as evidence of hormonal decline requiring replacement. On the other, you have guidelines so conservative that many people with genuine, symptomatic hormone deficiencies go untreated for years. Somewhere between these poles lies the territory where good clinical decision-making actually lives.

The reality is this: hormonal change is a universal feature of ageing, and some of those changes are clinically significant. The decline in sex hormones, adrenal hormones, and pituitary-driven growth signals contributes meaningfully to changes in body composition, bone density, cardiovascular risk, cognitive function, metabolic health, and quality of life. Understanding which of these changes matter, which ones warrant consideration of intervention, and under what circumstances, is genuinely important for anyone navigating the second half of life.

This chapter covers the major hormonal changes of ageing, their biological consequences, and the current evidence on when and how intervention may be appropriate. It is not a prescription — it is an honest, evidence-based framework for understanding a complex topic. Specific hormonal decisions must always be made in partnership with a doctor who can assess your individual circumstances, risk factors, and preferences.

The Hormonal Landscape of Ageing

Multiple hormonal systems change progressively with age. The most clinically significant involve four major axes: the gonadal (sex hormone) axis, the adrenal (stress and precursor hormone) axis, the somatotropic (growth hormone and IGF-1) axis, and the thyroid axis. Each declines at different rates, with different biological consequences, and each is influenced substantially by lifestyle factors — which is one reason why the same chronological age can correspond to vastly different hormonal profiles in different people.

A critical point before proceeding: hormonal decline in ageing is not uniformly pathological. Some degree of hormonal change is a normal feature of a long life. The biological question is whether a given individual's hormone levels have declined to a point where the benefits of correction outweigh the risks of intervention — a question that requires individual assessment, not population-level rules. The single most important thing you can do for your hormonal health as you age is invest in the lifestyle foundations covered in Part Two: sleep, exercise, nutrition, and stress management all have direct, measurable effects on hormone production and sensitivity.

Menopause: The Most Significant Hormonal Transition

Menopause — the cessation of ovarian function and the accompanying precipitous decline in oestrogen and progesterone — is the most abrupt and universal hormonal transition in human biology. Unlike the gradual hormone decline seen in men, menopause produces a rapid withdrawal of oestrogen that has consequences across virtually every physiological system: cardiovascular, skeletal, neurological, metabolic, and genitourinary.

The average age of menopause in Australia is 51 years, with perimenopause typically beginning in the mid-to-late forties. Symptoms during this transition include vasomotor symptoms (hot flushes, night sweats), sleep disruption, mood changes, brain fog, joint pain, reduced libido, and genitourinary changes. These are not merely inconvenient — they have real biological drivers and, for many women, significant impacts on work performance, relationships, and quality of life.

Beyond symptoms, the long-term health consequences of oestrogen loss are substantial. Cardiovascular disease risk increases markedly after menopause — not because menopause causes cardiovascular disease, but because oestrogen had been providing meaningful cardioprotection, and its withdrawal removes that protection. Bone mineral density declines at an accelerated rate in the first five to ten years after menopause, driving fracture risk. Metabolic health typically deteriorates, with shifts toward central adiposity, insulin resistance, and dyslipidaemia. Some evidence suggests the menopausal transition is also associated with acceleration of biological ageing as measured by epigenetic clocks.

The WHI Story and What It Actually Means

To understand the current state of menopausal hormone therapy (MHT), it helps to understand the history. In 2002, the Women's Health Initiative (WHI) study reported that hormone replacement therapy — specifically oral conjugated equine oestrogen combined with medroxyprogesterone acetate (MPA) — increased the risk of breast cancer, cardiovascular events, and stroke. The findings caused a massive, arguably panic-driven, collapse in MHT prescribing worldwide, with many women abruptly stopping treatment and many GPs becoming reluctant to prescribe it.

The subsequent two decades of analysis, re-examination, and new research have substantially modified the picture the WHI initially painted. Several critical issues have become clearer. First, the WHI population was older — the average participant was 63 years of age, a decade or more past menopause — not the women who stand to benefit most from MHT, which are those starting treatment within ten years of menopause onset. Second, the specific formulation used (oral conjugated equine oestrogen combined with synthetic progestogen MPA) is not the same as modern bioidentical preparations. Third, the absolute risk increases reported were small — fewer than ten additional events per 10,000 women — and were specific to that formulation, that population, and that route of administration.

> *"The timing hypothesis is now well-established: MHT initiated within ten years of menopause, or before age 60, has a meaningfully different and more favourable benefit-risk profile than treatment begun in older women."*

The Timing Hypothesis

The most important concept in modern MHT practice is the timing hypothesis: the biological effects of oestrogen on the cardiovascular system, brain, and bone depend critically on when treatment is initiated relative to the menopausal transition. Oestrogen has protective effects on a healthy, intact endothelium — the lining of blood vessels. Initiated in women within ten years of menopause or before age 60 years, MHT reduces all-cause mortality and cardiovascular disease risk. Initiated in older women with established atherosclerosis, the same therapy may have neutral or even adverse cardiovascular effects.

A comprehensive review published in Cancer Journal (2022) concluded that MHT initiated in women under 60 or within ten years of menopause significantly reduces all-cause mortality and cardiovascular disease — an effect that lipid-lowering therapy alone fails to achieve in women. The Danish Osteoporosis Prevention Trial — a randomised controlled trial in recently menopausal women aged 45 to 58 — found a 48 per cent reduction in risk of coronary heart disease in women receiving MHT compared to placebo. A 2024 meta-analysis and systematic review up to September 2025 (Cagnacci et al.) confirmed that MHT provides the most effective treatment for vasomotor symptoms, prevents early bone loss, and that early initiation with transdermal oestradiol is favoured when cardiometabolic or thrombotic risk is a concern.

The 2024 Lancet Diabetes and Endocrinology review explicitly proposed that the existing guidelines, which restrict MHT initiation to women within ten years of menopause or under 60, may be too conservative for women who remain symptomatic or at high fracture risk beyond those limits.

Bioidentical MHT: How Formulation Changes the Risk Picture

The timing hypothesis remains biologically valid with modern bioidentical formulations — but using regulated bioidentical hormones substantially reduces many of the specific risks that made the timing window so critical when the WHI was conducted. This distinction matters enormously in practice.

The timing hypothesis is fundamentally about the relationship between oestrogen and the endothelium — that principle does not change with formulation. What does change is the magnitude of the risks on either side of the equation. With transdermal oestradiol (patches, gels, or sprays), the first-pass liver effect is bypassed entirely, eliminating the coagulation factor surge that makes oral oestrogens increase venous thromboembolism (VTE) risk approximately two-fold. Multiple observational studies and meta-analyses confirm that transdermal oestradiol at standard doses carries no increased VTE risk compared to no treatment. Stroke risk is similarly more neutral with transdermal delivery than with oral preparations. Micronised progesterone — body-identical progesterone that is chemically and structurally identical to the progesterone the ovaries produce — does not carry the pro-thrombotic, pro-inflammatory, or mitogenic breast tissue effects of synthetic progestogens such as MPA. The combination of transdermal oestradiol and micronised progesterone therefore creates a substantially more favourable safety profile than the oral conjugated equine oestrogen plus MPA studied in the WHI, and the benefit-risk calculation is more favourable across a wider range of women and a broader time window than older guidelines based on WHI data might suggest.

One important distinction: the evidence and regulatory approval discussed here refers to pharmaceutical-grade, TGA-approved bioidentical preparations — transdermal oestradiol products (such as patches, gels, and sprays) and micronised progesterone capsules (such as Prometrium and Utrogestan) — not to custom-compounded bioidentical hormones dispensed by compounding pharmacies. Compounded preparations lack standardised dosing, quality control, and long-term safety data. The Menopause Society, Endocrine Society, ACOG, and the Royal Australian and New Zealand College of Obstetricians and Gynaecologists all advise against compounded bioidentical preparations in preference to regulated pharmaceutical products. This is a critical distinction that patients often miss when navigating the considerable online and social media noise around 'natural' or 'bioidentical' hormones.

Progesterone and the Brain: A Neurosteroid Story

One of the most compelling and underappreciated aspects of micronised progesterone is its role as a neurosteroid — a hormone produced not only by the ovaries but by the brain itself, acting directly on neural tissue. This distinguishes it fundamentally from synthetic progestogens, which do not share these neuroactive properties and in some cases actively undermine brain health.

The key mechanism runs through allopregnanolone — a potent metabolite of progesterone synthesised in the brain from cholesterol via progesterone. Allopregnanolone is a positive allosteric modulator of GABA-A receptors, the brain's principal inhibitory receptors, producing anxiolytic, pro-sleep, antidepressant, neuroprotective, and anticonvulsant effects. In practical terms, this helps explain why women taking micronised progesterone consistently report better sleep quality and reduced anxiety compared to those taking synthetic progestogens. These are not placebo effects — they reflect allopregnanolone's direct GABAergic action on the brain. Allopregnanolone is, in fact, so pharmacologically powerful that a synthetic analogue (brexanolone) was approved for the treatment of postpartum depression, with the mechanism being restoration of allopregnanolone signalling after its abrupt postpartum fall.

The neuroprotective case for progesterone is also mechanistically compelling. Progesterone receptors are widely distributed throughout the brain, particularly in the hippocampus, prefrontal cortex, and amygdala — regions critical for memory, executive function, and emotional regulation. Preclinical research consistently shows progesterone and allopregnanolone promote neurogenesis, support myelination, reduce neuroinflammation, and provide protection against excitotoxic and oxidative brain injury. Critically, allopregnanolone levels are reduced by over 50 per cent in the temporal cortex of Alzheimer's disease patients compared to cognitively intact controls — and this reduction correlates with Braak neuropathological stage, suggesting a direct relationship between allopregnanolone deficiency and neurodegeneration. Phase 2 clinical trials of allopregnanolone in Alzheimer's disease are currently underway (Bassani et al., 2023).

Crucially, MPA — the synthetic progestogen used in the WHI — has the opposite effect. Laboratory studies show MPA reduces both oestrogen receptor alpha and beta expression in neurons, actively blocks oestrogen-mediated neuroprotection, and suppresses BDNF (brain-derived neurotrophic factor) production. Natural progesterone does not carry these antagonistic properties. Some researchers now argue that the type of progestogen used in MHT is the most critical determinant of cognitive outcomes — more important than the type of oestrogen (Maki, 2012). This framing reframes the WHI dementia findings: the signal of harm may have been largely about MPA, not about hormone therapy itself.

A note of clinical honesty is warranted here: while the mechanistic and preclinical case for progesterone's neuroprotective role is strong, the direct evidence from human clinical trials for cognitive benefit from micronised progesterone in menopausal women is still emerging and not yet definitive. Small trials show mixed results, and the cognitive benefits seen in preclinical models have not yet been fully replicated in powered human trials. What is well established clinically is the sleep and anxiolytic benefit via allopregnanolone, the clear advantage over MPA in terms of not undermining brain health, and the growing case from observational and mechanistic research for neuroprotective potential. Women and their doctors should be aware of this emerging story, and should view the shift from synthetic progestogens to micronised progesterone as neurologically advantageous — while awaiting the outcome of ongoing clinical trials for more definitive evidence on dementia prevention.

MHT in Practice: Key Principles

For women considering or using MHT, the following principles reflect current best evidence:

- Initiation within ten years of menopause or before age 60 has the most favourable benefit-risk profile for most women, and should be considered the primary therapeutic window.

- Transdermal oestradiol (patches, gels, sprays) is preferred over oral oestrogen for women with any cardiovascular or thrombotic risk, as transdermal delivery avoids the first-pass liver effect that increases clotting factor production with oral preparations.

- Micronised progesterone (body-identical progesterone) is preferred over synthetic progestogens such as MPA when a progestogen is required for uterine protection, as it has a better cardiovascular and breast tissue safety profile.

- Local (vaginal) oestrogen for genitourinary symptoms carries minimal systemic absorption and essentially no systemic risk, and is appropriate for essentially any woman with GSM (genitourinary syndrome of menopause), including those who cannot or prefer not to use systemic MHT.

- Duration of treatment should be individualised — there is no universal 'five-year rule'. Many women benefit from continued treatment, and the decision to continue should be based on ongoing benefit-risk assessment rather than an arbitrary time limit.

- Breast cancer risk: the absolute increase in breast cancer risk with combined MHT using synthetic progestogens is small (fewer than ten additional cases per 10,000 women per year) and comparable to drinking one to two alcoholic drinks daily. Oestrogen-only therapy in women without a uterus is not associated with increased breast cancer risk. Critically, micronised progesterone appears neutral on breast tissue and does not carry the same risk signal as synthetic progestogens such as MPA — this is one of the most clinically significant advantages of the bioidentical formulation combination.

- All MHT decisions should be made in consultation with a doctor, incorporating individual risk factors, symptom burden, personal values, and preferences. A 'one size fits all' approach in either direction — universal prescribing or universal avoidance — is not consistent with current evidence.

Testosterone Decline in Men: Andropause and Its Consequences

Men do not undergo the abrupt hormonal withdrawal that characterises female menopause. Testosterone declines gradually in men from approximately the third decade of life onwards — at a rate of roughly one per cent per year for total testosterone and two per cent per year for free (biologically active) testosterone. By the age of 80, approximately 40 to 50 per cent of men have testosterone levels below those of normal healthy young individuals.

The biological consequences of testosterone decline — sometimes termed andropause or late-onset hypogonadism — include reduced libido, erectile dysfunction, decreased muscle mass and strength, increased visceral fat, reduced bone density, fatigue, low mood, and reduced cognitive function in some domains. These effects are real and well-documented, but they are also non-specific — many of these symptoms have other causes — and they overlap substantially with the effects of obesity, poor sleep, inactivity, and metabolic disease, all of which independently suppress testosterone.

This overlap is clinically important. A man in his fifties presenting with fatigue, reduced libido, and declining muscle mass might have genuinely low testosterone — or he might have sleep apnoea, depression, metabolic syndrome, or simply insufficient exercise. A testosterone measurement that comes back at the lower end of normal does not, by itself, indicate that testosterone replacement is indicated. The clinical picture must be considered as a whole.

The Evidence for TRT in Older Men

A landmark 2024 review published in the European Journal of Endocrinology — authored by researchers at the University of Melbourne and the University of Western Australia — synthesised findings from four recent large randomised controlled trials of testosterone therapy in middle-aged and older men with low or low-normal testosterone and no identifiable pituitary-testicular axis pathology (Grossmann et al., 2024). The conclusions were nuanced and clinically important:

- Testosterone therapy produced modest but clinically meaningful benefits in self-reported energy, mood, sexual function, and satisfaction.

- In men at high risk of or with newly diagnosed type 2 diabetes, testosterone therapy combined with a lifestyle programme reversed or reduced incident diabetes.

- Modest improvements in objectively assessed muscle strength and walking distance were demonstrated.

- Bone density and strength increased, though fracture reduction was not demonstrated.

- No significant increase in myocardial infarction, stroke, or prostate cancer risk was seen over the trial periods.

- The most common significant adverse effect was erythrocytosis (elevated red blood cell count), requiring monitoring.

A 2025 systematic review confirmed that TRT consistently improved sexual desire, erectile function, lean body mass, bone mineral density, insulin sensitivity, and vitality in men with confirmed hypogonadism, with a favourable safety profile under structured monitoring. The review reinforced that benefits are most clearly seen in men with genuinely low testosterone, not merely at the lower end of the normal range.

The current consensus position of the Endocrine Society is that testosterone therapy should be offered on an individualised basis to men over 65 with symptoms or conditions consistent with testosterone deficiency and consistently low testosterone levels. Widespread prescribing of testosterone to all older men with age-related decline in testosterone is not currently justified by the evidence, and should be distinguished from treatment of true hypogonadism.

Optimising Testosterone Without TRT: What Lifestyle Can Do

Before considering pharmacological testosterone replacement, the lifestyle levers that support testosterone production deserve serious attention. Sleep deprivation acutely suppresses testosterone — men who sleep five hours rather than eight hours have testosterone levels equivalent to someone ten years older. Resistance training is one of the most powerful natural testosterone stimulants available. Reducing visceral adiposity — through exercise and dietary improvement — independently raises testosterone, often substantially, in overweight men. Chronic stress and cortisol excess directly suppress gonadotropins and Leydig cell function. Alcohol, in quantity, impairs testosterone synthesis. Optimising these factors before or alongside considering TRT is both good medicine and good sense.

DHEA and Adrenopause: The Forgotten Hormone

Dehydroepiandrosterone (DHEA) and its sulphated form DHEA-S are the most abundant steroid hormones in circulation. Produced primarily by the adrenal glands, DHEA serves as a precursor for the synthesis of both oestrogens and androgens in peripheral tissues, and has independent biological effects on immune function, metabolic health, bone density, and potentially brain function. DHEA peaks around age 25 and then declines at approximately two per cent per year, so that by age 70, circulating levels are only 20 to 30 per cent of peak values.

This dramatic, universal decline — termed adrenopause — is one of the most consistent hormonal features of ageing. Whether it is a cause of age-related decline or simply a marker of it remains contested. Observational studies consistently link low DHEA-S levels to increased mortality, frailty, cardiovascular disease, and cognitive impairment in older adults. Whether supplementing DHEA meaningfully reverses these associations is less clear, with trial evidence showing modest improvements in wellbeing, some benefit for bone density in women, and mixed results for other outcomes. DHEA replacement is more established in the treatment of adrenal insufficiency (where the adrenal glands fail to produce adequate hormones) than in normal ageing.

DHEA is not regulated as a prescription medicine in Australia and is available as a supplement, though it is a scheduled substance and its unmonitored use raises the same questions about appropriate dosing and potential adverse effects as any hormone precursor. For those interested in DHEA, a clinical assessment of actual DHEA-S levels and guidance from a practitioner experienced in hormonal medicine is strongly recommended over self-directed supplementation.

The Somatotropic Axis: Growth Hormone, IGF-1, and Ageing

Growth hormone (GH) is secreted in pulses throughout the day and night by the pituitary gland, with the largest pulses occurring during slow-wave sleep. Its principal downstream mediator is insulin-like growth factor 1 (IGF-1), produced primarily in the liver. GH and IGF-1 drive growth and anabolism in early life — and their declining levels in middle and later life contribute to reduced muscle mass, increased body fat, reduced bone density, and diminished exercise capacity. This age-related decline in the GH/IGF-1 axis is termed somatopause.

The relationship between GH, IGF-1, and longevity is genuinely complex and somewhat counterintuitive. In animal models — particularly in mice — reduced GH signalling is consistently associated with significantly longer lifespans and better healthspan. Mice with genetic deficiency or resistance to GH live dramatically longer than normal mice. In humans, individuals with hereditary GH deficiency or resistance show reduced rates of age-related disease. Yet paradoxically, recombinant GH treatment in middle-aged and older adults with naturally declining GH levels can produce beneficial effects on body composition and quality of life in the short to medium term. The nuance appears to be that chronic excessive GH (as in acromegaly) accelerates ageing, while absence of GH from birth is protective — and that the physiological decline of middle age occupies a different territory than either extreme.

Recombinant GH therapy for age-related somatopause is not recommended or approved in Australia or most Western countries outside of specific clinical indications (such as adult GH deficiency from pituitary pathology). The evidence for long-term safety and benefit in otherwise healthy older adults is insufficient to justify its use, and the risks — including glucose intolerance, fluid retention, and potential cancer risk — are not trivial. The most effective approach to supporting GH secretion is, again, lifestyle-based: deep sleep (when most GH is secreted), resistance and high-intensity exercise, intermittent fasting, and maintaining a healthy body composition all support endogenous GH pulsatility.

Thyroid Function: The Metabolic Regulator

The thyroid gland produces hormones (principally thyroxine, T4, and triiodothyronine, T3) that regulate metabolic rate across virtually every organ system. Thyroid dysfunction becomes increasingly common with age — hypothyroidism (underactive thyroid) affects approximately 5 to 10 per cent of adults over 65 in Australia, with subclinical hypothyroidism (mildly elevated TSH with normal free thyroid hormones) being considerably more common, particularly in women.

The symptoms of hypothyroidism — fatigue, weight gain, cold intolerance, constipation, brain fog, dry skin, low mood — overlap extensively with many other conditions of midlife and beyond, which is one reason it is frequently missed. A simple blood test measuring TSH (thyroid stimulating hormone) and free T4 and T3 provides an accurate and inexpensive screen. Overt hypothyroidism in symptomatic patients is clearly treatable and the benefits of levothyroxine replacement are well established.

Subclinical hypothyroidism — defined as an elevated TSH with normal free T4 — occupies a more contested space. Whether treating subclinical hypothyroidism in older adults improves outcomes is genuinely unclear, with some trials showing benefit in younger patients but neutral or mixed results in older adults. Current guidance from Australian endocrinologists generally supports treating symptomatic subclinical hypothyroidism in younger people but recommends individualised decision-making in older adults, particularly since mildly elevated TSH in older age may be a physiological adaptation rather than a pathological process.

For anyone over 45 who has not had thyroid function checked recently, a TSH and free T4/T3 through their GP is a low-cost, high-value assessment. Thyroid function also provides context for other hormonal evaluations — thyroid dysfunction can mimic and confound symptoms that might otherwise be attributed to sex hormone decline.

Hormonal Changes of Ageing: A Clinical Overview

Hormone / Axis	Pattern of Decline	Key Consequences	When to Consider Intervention
Oestrogen / Progesterone (women)	Abrupt at menopause (~51 yrs); perimenopause from mid-40s	Vasomotor symptoms, bone loss, CV risk increase, metabolic shift, GSM	Symptomatic peri/post-menopause; within 10 years of menopause or before age 60 generally favoured
Testosterone (men)	Gradual: ~1%/yr total T, ~2%/yr free T from 3rd decade	Muscle loss, fat gain, reduced libido, fatigue, low mood, bone loss	Confirmed hypogonadism with symptoms (total T <10 nmol/L + symptoms); lifestyle optimisation first
DHEA / DHEA-S	~2%/yr from age 25; 70-80% lost by age 70	Reduced precursor for sex hormones; possible fatigue, immune effects, bone effects	Adrenal insufficiency (established indication); ageing per se — evidence limited and mixed
Growth Hormone / IGF-1	Progressive decline from 3rd decade; mostly nocturnal secretion reduced	Muscle and fat composition changes, reduced exercise capacity, bone effects	Pituitary GH deficiency (pathological); age-related somatopause — not currently indicated

Hormone / Axis	Pattern of Decline	Key Consequences	When to Consider Intervention
Thyroid (T3/T4)	Prevalence of hypothyroidism rises with age; subclinical hypothyroidism common	Fatigue, weight gain, brain fog, cold intolerance, low mood	Overt hypothyroidism: treat. Subclinical: individualised, especially in older adults

~51 yrs average age of menopause in Australia; perimenopause typically begins mid-to-late 40s

~1-2%/yr rate of testosterone decline in men from the 3rd decade; free T declines faster than total T

10 years the 'timing window' within which MHT initiation has the most favourable benefit-risk profile

5-10% prevalence of hypothyroidism in Australians over 65; subclinical hypothyroidism is considerably more common

The Lifestyle Foundation: What You Can Do Before Considering Hormones

The single most important message of this chapter is that hormonal health in midlife is substantially modifiable through lifestyle — and that addressing these factors before or alongside any pharmacological intervention is both evidence-based and often remarkably effective. The following are the lifestyle factors with the strongest evidence for supporting hormonal health across the board:

- **Sleep:** Growth hormone is predominantly secreted during slow-wave sleep. Testosterone is produced and restored during sleep. Cortisol — which suppresses sex hormone production — is regulated through sleep quality. The hormonal consequences of chronic poor sleep are substantial and well-documented. Protecting sleep quality, as discussed in Chapter Four, is one of the highest-leverage hormonal interventions available.

- **Resistance training:** Resistance exercise is the most powerful natural stimulus for testosterone and growth hormone secretion. It also improves insulin sensitivity (which in turn improves hormonal signalling across multiple axes), increases muscle mass and bone density, and reduces visceral fat. The evidence for resistance training as a cornerstone of hormonal health in midlife and beyond is overwhelming.

- **Reducing visceral adiposity:** Visceral fat is metabolically active and pro-inflammatory. Aromatase in adipose tissue converts testosterone to oestrogen in both men and women, which can contribute to oestrogen excess relative to testosterone in overweight men. Visceral fat also promotes insulin resistance, which impairs the hormonal milieu across multiple axes. Reducing central adiposity through diet and exercise independently improves testosterone, insulin sensitivity, and the overall hormonal environment.

- **Stress management:** Chronic cortisol excess from sustained HPA activation directly suppresses gonadotropin-releasing hormone (GnRH) at the hypothalamus, reducing LH and FSH, and thereby suppressing gonadal hormone production in both sexes. Managing chronic stress, as discussed in Chapter Seven, is therefore also a hormonal health strategy.

- **Nutrition:** Adequate dietary fat intake supports steroid hormone synthesis (all steroid hormones are derived from cholesterol). Micronutrient status — particularly zinc, magnesium, and vitamin D — affects testosterone production and hormonal receptor sensitivity. Avoiding excessive calorie restriction, which suppresses the hypothalamic-pituitary-gonadal axis, is relevant for both men and women.

- **Alcohol and toxin avoidance:** Alcohol impairs testosterone synthesis and increases aromatisation, directly lowering testosterone and raising oestrogen in men. Several environmental endocrine disruptors — found in plastics, pesticides, and personal care products — may affect hormonal function through oestrogen mimicry or androgen antagonism. Reducing unnecessary chemical exposures is a reasonable precaution with minimal downside.

Getting Your Hormones Assessed: A Practical Guide

Understanding your hormonal status begins with testing. In Australia, most of the relevant assessments are available through your GP and covered under Medicare for appropriate clinical indications. The following provides a practical guide to what to ask about and why:

Test	What It Measures	Clinical Relevance
TSH + Free T4/T3	Thyroid-stimulating hormone and free thyroxine	First-line thyroid screen. Elevated TSH suggests hypothyroidism; suppressed TSH suggests hyperthyroidism or over-replacement.
Total + Free Testosterone (men)	Total and bioavailable testosterone; ideally with SHBG	Assess morning fasting sample. At least two measurements needed to confirm hypogonadism. Free T more informative than total T.
FSH + LH	Follicle-stimulating and luteinising hormones	Elevated in primary gonadal failure; helps distinguish gonadal from pituitary causes of low sex hormones.

Test	What It Measures	Clinical Relevance
Oestradiol (women)	Circulating oestrogen	Most useful in perimenopause alongside FSH. Single measurements less informative than clinical picture in reproductive years.
DHEA-S	Adrenal androgen precursor	Marker of adrenal function and adrenopause. Low levels correlate with frailty and mortality in population studies.
IGF-1	Downstream marker of GH secretion	Useful indicator of somatotropic axis function. Low for age suggests relative GH deficiency.
Prolactin	Pituitary hormone	Elevated prolactin suppresses sex hormones in both sexes. Important to exclude if low testosterone or oestrogen found.
Cortisol (morning)	Adrenal stress hormone	Chronic elevation suppresses sex hormones. Morning sample provides baseline; salivary cortisol patterns more informative for chronic stress assessment.

A note on 'comprehensive hormone panels' from direct-to-consumer or online providers: while the democratisation of testing is generally positive, results without clinical context are often more confusing than illuminating. A testosterone result at the lower end of normal range does not tell you whether intervention is appropriate without knowing the clinical picture, symptom burden, lifestyle factors, and individual risk profile. Test with a clinician, not just a lab.

Hormones in Perspective

Hormonal health is one dimension of a complex, interconnected biological system. No hormone operates in isolation, and no hormonal intervention can substitute for the foundational lifestyle practices that support the entire system. Sleep, exercise, nutrition, and stress management are not just complementary to hormonal health — in many cases, they are the primary determinants of it.

At the same time, this chapter should make clear that for people with genuine hormonal deficiencies, appropriately targeted and monitored intervention can make a meaningful difference to healthspan. Menopausal hormone therapy initiated at the right time and in the right formulation is one of the most effective preventive health interventions available to women in midlife. Testosterone therapy for men with confirmed symptomatic hypogonadism, under appropriate clinical supervision, is a legitimate and evidence-based option. Thyroid replacement in overt hypothyroidism is essentially uncontroversial.

The path through this landscape requires a doctor who understands both the evidence and the individual in front of them. If you feel your hormonal health concerns are not being adequately addressed, seeking a second opinion from a GP with a special interest in endocrinology or integrative medicine, or from an endocrinologist or menopause specialist, is entirely reasonable. In Australia, the Australasian Menopause Society and the Endocrine Society of Australia both maintain directories of practitioners with relevant expertise.

Chapter Summary

- Multiple hormonal axes decline with age: the gonadal axis (oestrogen/testosterone), adrenal axis (DHEA), somatotropic axis (GH/IGF-1), and thyroid. Each has different biological consequences and different evidence for intervention.

- Menopause is the most significant hormonal transition in human biology, producing rapid oestrogen withdrawal with consequences for cardiovascular, skeletal, metabolic, neurological, and genitourinary health.

- The timing hypothesis is now well-supported: MHT initiated within ten years of menopause or before age 60 significantly reduces all-cause mortality and cardiovascular disease. Transdermal oestradiol and micronised progesterone are the preferred modern formulations — and their substantially better safety profile (no VTE increase, neutral breast tissue effects, better cardiovascular profile) means the benefit-risk calculation is more favourable across a wider window than older WHI-based guidelines suggest.

- Breast cancer risk with combined MHT using synthetic progestogens is small in absolute terms and formulation-dependent. Oestrogen-only therapy carries essentially no increased breast risk. Micronised progesterone appears neutral on breast tissue — a key advantage over synthetic progestogens. Regulated pharmaceutical-grade bioidentical preparations (TGA-approved transdermal oestradiol and micronised progesterone) are preferable to compounded bioidentical preparations, which lack standardised dosing and safety data. Micronised progesterone is also a neurosteroid whose metabolite allopregnanolone supports sleep, reduces anxiety, and may protect brain health — in direct contrast to MPA, which blocks oestrogen-mediated neuroprotection and suppresses BDNF.

- Testosterone declines gradually in men at ~1–2%/year from the third decade. Consequences include muscle loss, fat gain, reduced libido, fatigue, and bone loss. TRT in men with confirmed symptomatic hypogonadism offers modest but meaningful benefits with acceptable safety when monitored appropriately.

- Lifestyle is the most important modifiable determinant of hormonal health: sleep quality, resistance training, reducing visceral fat, stress management, and avoiding alcohol excess all directly support testosterone, GH, and the overall hormonal milieu.

- Thyroid dysfunction affects 5–10% of Australians over 65 and is easily screened with a TSH and free T4/T3. Overt hypothyroidism is clearly treatable; subclinical hypothyroidism in older adults requires individualised decision-making.

- All hormonal intervention decisions should be made in partnership with a clinician who can assess individual risk factors, symptom burden, and preferences. Testing without clinical context is rarely sufficient for sound decision-making.

References

Grossmann, M., Anawalt, B. D., & Yeap, B. B. (2024). Testosterone therapy in older men: clinical implications of recent landmark trials. European Journal of Endocrinology, 191(1), R22–R31. https://doi.org/10.1093/ejendo/lvae071

Cagnacci, A., et al. (2025). Menopausal hormone therapy — risks, benefits and emerging options: a narrative review. International Journal of Molecular Sciences, 26(22), 11098. https://doi.org/10.3390/ijms262211098

Hodis, H. N., & Mack, W. J. (2022). Menopausal hormone replacement therapy and reduction of all-cause mortality and cardiovascular disease: it's about time and timing. Cancer Journal, 28(3), 208–223. https://pmc.ncbi.nlm.nih.gov/articles/PMC9178928/

Rees, M., et al. (2023). Global consensus recommendations on menopause in the workplace: a European Menopause and Andropause Society (EMAS) position statement. Maturitas. https://doi.org/10.1016/j.maturitas.2021.10.005

Manson, J. E., & Bassuk, S. S. (2024). Is it time to revisit the recommendations for initiation of menopausal hormone therapy? Lancet Diabetes and Endocrinology. https://doi.org/10.1016/S2213-8587(24)00270-5

Cappola, A. R., et al. (2023). Hormones and aging: an Endocrine Society Scientific Statement. Journal of Clinical Endocrinology and Metabolism.

Saad, F., et al. (2025). Testosterone replacement therapy in men aged 50 and above: a narrative review.

PMC.
https://pmc.ncbi.nlm.nih.gov/articles/PMC12535424/

Bhasin, S., et al. (2021). Testosterone replacement in aging men: an evidence-based patient-centric perspective. Journal of Clinical Investigation, 131(4). https://pmc.ncbi.nlm.nih.gov/articles/PMC7880314/

Giordano, R., et al. (2023). Age-related hormonal changes and their impact on health status and lifespan. Aging and Disease. https://pmc.ncbi.nlm.nih.gov/articles/PMC10187696/

Giannoulis, M. G., et al. (2012). Hormone replacement therapy and physical function in healthy older men. Time to talk hormones? Endocrine Reviews, 33(3), 314–377.

Chapter Ten

The Gut-Longevity Axis

*How the trillions of organisms living in
your gut shape your ageing trajectory
— and what you can do about it*

There are more microbial cells in your gut than there are human cells in your entire body. The collective genome of these organisms — your gut microbiome — contains over a hundred times more genes than the human genome. This is not a minor biological footnote. It represents a parallel biological system, living inside us, that has co-evolved with human physiology over millions of years and is now emerging as one of the most significant determinants of how we age.

The gut microbiome is not simply a digestive accessory. It is an endocrine organ, producing hundreds of bioactive compounds. It is an immune regulator, calibrating the balance between inflammatory and anti-inflammatory signals throughout the body. It is a neurological communicant, sending signals to the brain via the vagus nerve, the enteric nervous system, and the bloodstream. And it is, increasingly, understood to be a modifiable determinant of biological ageing — one that is being actively reshaped, for better or worse, by every food choice, lifestyle factor, and medication you encounter.

This chapter explores the gut-longevity axis: what the research tells us about how the microbiome changes with age, how those changes contribute to disease and accelerated biological ageing, and — most practically — what you can do to cultivate a gut environment that supports your healthspan.

The Ageing Microbiome: What Changes and Why It Matters

The gut microbiome is not static. It changes profoundly across the lifespan, shaped by diet, medications, illness, geographic location, and the ageing process itself. In broad terms, a healthy adult gut is characterised by high microbial diversity — a rich community of hundreds of different bacterial species working in dynamic balance. What consistently happens as we age is a decline in this diversity, a reduction in beneficial bacteria, and an increase in potentially pro-inflammatory species.

A systematic review of 27 human studies spanning the full age range found that older adults with higher microbial diversity — particularly the oldest-old — had distinct microbiome profiles associated with better health outcomes. The most consistently reported age-related changes include a decline in Faecalibacterium prausnitzii and Lachnospiraceae (key butyrate-producing species with anti-inflammatory properties), and increases in more opportunistic taxa. In parallel, short-chain fatty acid production — the microbiome's primary currency for gut health and systemic inflammation control — tends to decline with age in most populations (Badal et al., 2020).

Centenarian studies have added a particularly compelling dimension to this picture. Multiple large cohort studies, including a comprehensive metagenomic analysis of 1,156 faecal samples published in 2024, have found that extremely long-lived people maintain higher microbial diversity than younger older adults, with enrichment in beneficial species including several not typically found in younger cohorts. Mendelian randomisation analysis in this study suggested a potential causal relationship between certain microbial signatures and longevity. Transplanting faecal microbiota from long-lived donors into aged mice has been shown to increase microbial diversity, reduce neuroinflammation markers, and extend healthy lifespan in animal models — providing some of the most compelling causal evidence to date.

"Centenarians maintain a more 'youthful' gut microbiome than younger old adults — with higher diversity, enriched beneficial taxa, and greater SCFA production capacity. Some researchers now propose the microbiome as an emerging tenth hallmark of ageing."

The bidirectional relationship is equally important. The microbiome influences ageing, but ageing also changes the microbiome. Reduced gastric acid secretion with age impairs the hostile environment that normally limits bacterial overgrowth. Reduced gut motility changes transit time and fermentation patterns. Polypharmacy — the simultaneous use of multiple medications common in older adults — significantly disrupts microbial composition, with antibiotics, proton pump inhibitors, metformin, and many other drugs each producing characteristic microbiome perturbations. Reduced dietary variety and total food intake in older adults reduces the diversity of substrate available for microbial fermentation. The result is a progressive decline in the gut environment that both reflects and accelerates broader biological ageing.

How the Gut Microbiome Affects Your Biology: The Key Pathways

Short-Chain Fatty Acids: The Microbiome's Master Metabolites

Short-chain fatty acids (SCFAs) — primarily butyrate, propionate, and acetate — are produced when gut bacteria ferment dietary fibre. They represent the primary language through which the microbiome communicates with the rest of the body, and their decline with age is one of the most consequential features of the ageing gut.

Butyrate is the most studied of the three. It is the primary energy source for colonocytes (the cells lining the colon), and without adequate butyrate production, colonocyte function deteriorates, gut barrier integrity weakens, and the risk of both inflammatory bowel conditions and colorectal cancer increases. Beyond the gut, butyrate crosses the blood-brain barrier, inhibits histone deacetylases (HDAC inhibition being an epigenetic mechanism with anti-inflammatory and anti-cancer effects), promotes autophagy, and reduces systemic inflammation. It activates G-protein coupled receptors on immune cells throughout the body, producing consistently anti-inflammatory effects. Propionate regulates cholesterol synthesis and glucose metabolism. Acetate travels through the portal circulation to the liver and plays roles in lipid and cholesterol metabolism.

The key dietary determinant of SCFA production is fibre — specifically diverse, fermentable dietary fibre from vegetables, legumes, whole grains, and fruit. When dietary fibre intake falls, SCFA production falls. When dietary diversity falls, microbial diversity falls, reducing the range of fermentation products. This is one of the most direct mechanisms through which the dietary patterns discussed in Chapter Six translate into microbiome-mediated health effects.

Gut Barrier Integrity and Leaky Gut

The gut barrier — the single-cell-thick layer of epithelial cells that separates the contents of the gut from the bloodstream — is one of the most important and most frequently underappreciated structures in the body. When intact, it allows selective absorption of nutrients while blocking bacterial products, endotoxins, and other immune-activating materials from entering circulation. When this barrier is compromised — a condition colloquially called 'leaky gut' and more precisely termed increased intestinal permeability — bacterial lipopolysaccharide (LPS) and other microbial products enter the bloodstream and trigger a chronic, low-grade systemic inflammatory response.

This process, known as metabolic endotoxaemia, is now recognised as a significant contributor to inflammageing — the chronic low-grade inflammation that drives virtually every age-related disease from cardiovascular disease to dementia. High-fat, low-fibre diets, alcohol, chronic stress, NSAIDs, and the progressive microbiome changes of ageing all contribute to increased intestinal permeability. Conversely, adequate butyrate production (requiring adequate fibre intake and butyrate-producing bacteria) is one of the primary drivers of tight junction protein expression and gut barrier maintenance.

The Gut-Brain Axis

The connection between gut microbiome composition and brain health is one of the fastest-moving areas of biomedical research. The gut-brain axis is a bidirectional communication network linking the enteric nervous system (the '"second brain" of the gut, with around 500 million neurons), the vagus nerve, the immune system, and the bloodstream. Through these channels, the microbiome influences mood, cognition, stress responses, and the risk of neurodegenerative disease in ways that were not recognised a decade ago.

The mechanisms are multiple and reinforcing. Gut bacteria produce approximately 90 per cent of the body's serotonin and significant proportions of other neurotransmitters and neuromodulators. SCFAs, as already discussed, cross the blood-brain barrier and directly modulate neuroinflammation, microglial activity, and neurogenesis. Gut dysbiosis is consistently associated with neuroinflammation — the persistent low-grade inflammation of neural tissue that is a major driver of cognitive decline and neurodegeneration. Dysbiotic bacterial species can produce bacterial amyloid proteins that may cross-seed misfolding of host proteins like alpha-synuclein (relevant to Parkinson's disease) and amyloid-beta (relevant to Alzheimer's disease).

A landmark 2024 study published in Molecular Psychiatry followed 268 older adults with varying cognitive and depressive symptoms, with 70 participants followed for two years. The study found that microbiome composition not only reflected current cognitive function and depressive symptoms but predicted future cognitive decline and depression over the follow-up period — a finding with significant implications for early intervention. Alzheimer's disease is now consistently associated with reduced microbial diversity, lower levels of anti-inflammatory genera like Faecalibacterium, and elevated levels of pro-inflammatory taxa.

The Gut-Immune Axis and Inflammageing

The gut houses approximately 70 per cent of the body's immune tissue. The relationship between the microbiome and immune function is not incidental — the immune system largely learns from, and is calibrated by, microbial exposure throughout life. A diverse, healthy microbiome trains immune tolerance, reduces inappropriate inflammatory responses, and supports the regulatory T cell populations that prevent the immune system from attacking the body's own tissues.

Dysbiosis and reduced microbial diversity are now recognised as drivers of immunosenescence (the age-related decline in immune function) and inflammageing. The reduced SCFA production that accompanies gut ageing means reduced HDAC inhibition in immune cells, less regulatory T cell induction, and a progressive shift toward pro-inflammatory immune phenotypes. This is one of the key mechanistic links between gut health and the accelerated biological ageing described throughout this book.

100+ times more genes in the gut microbiome than in the human genome — the microbiome is a parallel biological operating system

90% of the body's serotonin is produced in the gut, with microbiome composition influencing production and neurotransmitter signalling

~70% of the body's immune tissue is in the gut — the microbiome is the primary calibrator of immune function throughout life

5.9 yrs accuracy with which machine-learning analysis of microbiome composition can predict a person's chronological age

Supporting Your Gut Microbiome: What the Evidence Supports

The microbiome is exquisitely sensitive to diet, lifestyle, and environmental factors. This sensitivity is both the problem — in a modern food environment dominated by ultra-processed foods, low fibre intake, and frequent antibiotic exposure — and the opportunity. No other biological system covered in this book responds as rapidly or as meaningfully to dietary intervention as the gut microbiome. Studies consistently show measurable changes in microbiome composition within days of dietary change. This makes it one of the highest-leverage areas for practical intervention.

Dietary Fibre: The Single Most Important Factor

Dietary fibre is the most important dietary determinant of gut microbiome health. It is the substrate for SCFA production, the primary driver of microbial diversity, and the critical input that keeps butyrate-producing bacteria fed and functional. The recommended intake in Australia is 25 to 30 grams per day; the average Australian consumes significantly less. Most people who are not specifically trying to increase fibre intake fall short of even the lower end of this range.

Not all fibre is equal from a microbiome perspective. Fermentable fibre — particularly prebiotic fibre including inulin, fructooligosaccharides, beta-glucan, and resistant starch — preferentially feeds beneficial bacteria. Rich sources include legumes (lentils, chickpeas, beans), Jerusalem artichokes, onions, garlic, leeks, asparagus, oats, barley, green bananas, and cooked-and-cooled potatoes and rice (the cooling process increases resistant starch content). Diversity of fibre sources drives diversity of microbiome composition — this is why eating a wide variety of plant foods matters beyond just meeting a gram target.

The practical message from the American Gut Project — the largest citizen science microbiome study to date — was striking: people who ate 30 or more different plant species per week had significantly greater microbiome diversity than those who ate fewer than 10. This '30 plants' concept has become a practical shorthand for supporting microbial diversity, and it is worth keeping in mind as a goal rather than a rigid prescription.

Fermented Foods

Fermented foods — yoghurt, kefir, sauerkraut, kimchi, miso, tempeh, and kombucha — contain live microorganisms that can transiently colonise the gut and produce beneficial effects on microbial composition and immune function. A 2021 randomised controlled trial from Stanford published in Cell found that a diet high in fermented foods increased microbiome diversity and reduced markers of immune activation over ten weeks — more effectively than a high-fibre diet alone in that study's participants. While the microorganisms from fermented foods do not typically establish permanent residence, their transient presence and metabolic activity appear to produce measurable benefits.

Fermented foods are not magic, and the evidence base for specific health claims attached to individual products is highly variable. But incorporating a variety of fermented foods regularly — particularly traditional fermented dairy products and lacto-fermented vegetables — is a low-risk, culturally familiar, and evidence-consistent approach to supporting gut microbiome health.

Mediterranean and Plant-Rich Dietary Patterns

The broader dietary patterns associated with healthspan — particularly the Mediterranean dietary pattern covered in Chapter Six — are also the patterns most consistently associated with higher microbiome diversity, greater SCFA production, and lower inflammatory markers. The two stories are deeply intertwined: the health benefits of Mediterranean eating are at least partly mediated through microbiome pathways. This is not coincidental — the traditional Mediterranean diet was high in diverse plant foods, legumes, fermented dairy, and whole grains long before anyone understood what the microbiome was.

Reducing Microbiome-Damaging Exposures

Supporting gut health is not only about what you add — it is equally about reducing the exposures that damage the microbiome. The most important include:

- **Antibiotics:** Antibiotics are the most potent disruptors of the gut microbiome, producing massive shifts in composition that can persist for months to years after a single course. This is not an argument against using antibiotics when genuinely needed — they save lives and must be taken when indicated. But it is an argument for avoiding unnecessary courses, completing courses as prescribed (incomplete courses favour resistant strains), and considering targeted probiotic support during and after antibiotic treatment.

- **Ultra-processed foods:** As discussed in Chapter Six, UPFs are low in the fermentable fibre that gut bacteria need, high in additives (emulsifiers, artificial sweeteners, preservatives) that directly disrupt the gut barrier and microbial composition, and associated with reduced microbiome diversity. This is one of the key biological mechanisms through which UPF consumption drives disease.

- **Proton pump inhibitors (PPIs):** PPIs are among the most widely prescribed medications in Australia and significantly alter gut microbiome composition by reducing gastric acidity. When genuinely indicated for conditions like Barrett's oesophagus or peptic ulcer disease, their benefits outweigh their risks. However, many Australians are taking PPIs for symptoms that could be managed with dietary change and lifestyle modification. A conversation with your GP about whether long-term PPI use is still necessary is worthwhile.

- **Excessive alcohol:** Alcohol disrupts gut barrier integrity, promotes dysbiosis, and increases LPS translocation. The dose-response relationship is clear: more alcohol means more gut damage. Reducing alcohol intake has measurable effects on gut barrier function within weeks.

- **Chronic stress:** The gut-brain axis runs in both directions. Chronic stress and cortisol elevation disrupt gut motility, reduce secretory IgA (the gut's primary immune defence), and promote dysbiosis. Managing stress, as discussed in Chapter Seven, is also managing gut health.

Exercise

Regular physical activity has independent effects on gut microbiome composition that go beyond its dietary context. Multiple studies in both animals and humans show that exercise increases microbial diversity, increases the abundance of butyrate-producing bacteria, and improves gut barrier integrity. The mechanisms include improved gut motility, reduced inflammatory markers, and direct effects on immune-microbiome interactions. These benefits appear to be partially independent of dietary changes — people who exercise more tend to have healthier gut microbiomes even when dietary differences are accounted for.

Probiotics and Prebiotics: What the Evidence Actually Shows

The probiotic supplement market is enormous and largely ahead of the science. Most over-the-counter probiotic products contain strains that have limited evidence for specific clinical outcomes in healthy adults, at doses that may be insufficient to produce lasting microbiome changes. This does not mean probiotics are useless — specific strains have demonstrated efficacy for specific clinical conditions including antibiotic-associated diarrhoea, irritable bowel syndrome, and some inflammatory bowel conditions — but the evidence for non-specific 'gut health' claims in healthy people is weaker than marketing suggests.

Prebiotic supplements (fibre-based products designed to feed beneficial bacteria) have a somewhat stronger evidence base for supporting microbiome composition than probiotic supplements in otherwise healthy people, since they address the fundamental substrate question rather than trying to introduce exogenous organisms. However, food-based prebiotic fibre — from the legumes, vegetables, and whole grains described above — is preferable to supplemental prebiotic fibre where achievable, for the same reasons that whole foods are generally preferable to supplements across nutrition.

For specific clinical situations — after antibiotic treatment, during and after gastrointestinal illness, for IBS, or for documented gut dysbiosis — targeted probiotic therapy guided by a clinician with expertise in gastrointestinal health is reasonable and may be beneficial. Self-directed probiotic supplementation as a general anti-ageing strategy is less well supported.

A Practical Gut Health Framework

Strategy	Practical Application	Evidence Level
Increase dietary fibre	Aim for 25–30g/day from diverse sources. Include legumes, vegetables, whole grains, fruit, nuts and seeds daily.	Strong — primary determinant of SCFA production and microbial diversity
Eat 30+ plant species weekly	Count every plant food: herbs, spices, teas, and fruit count. Diversity drives microbial diversity.	Strong — American Gut Project data (10,000+ participants)
Include fermented foods	Daily serve of yoghurt, kefir, sauerkraut, kimchi, or miso. Variety is better than large quantities of one type.	Moderate — RCT evidence for diversity increase and immune benefits
Minimise ultra-processed foods	UPFs displace fibre, contain microbiome-disrupting additives, and are associated with reduced diversity and increased intestinal permeability.	Strong — consistent across large cohort studies
Exercise regularly	Even moderate aerobic and resistance exercise increases butyrate-producing bacteria and microbiome diversity.	Moderate-strong — consistent findings across human and animal studies

Strategy	Practical Application	Evidence Level
Reduce unnecessary antibiotic use	Take when indicated; avoid unnecessary courses. Consider probiotic support during and after treatment.	Strong — antibiotics are the most potent microbiome disruptors available
Manage stress	Chronic stress disrupts gut motility, reduces secretory IgA, and promotes dysbiosis. Stress management is gut health.	Moderate — consistent mechanistic and observational evidence
Limit alcohol	Alcohol increases intestinal permeability and promotes dysbiosis in a dose-dependent manner. Any reduction helps.	Strong — dose-response relationship well established
Review PPIs if long-term	If taking PPIs without clear ongoing indication, discuss with GP. De-prescribing where appropriate reduces microbiome disruption.	Moderate — PPIs produce consistent microbiome alterations

Your Gut as a Long-Term Investment

The gut microbiome occupies a remarkable position in the biology of ageing: it is simultaneously one of the most powerful determinants of healthspan and one of the most practically modifiable. Unlike your genetics or your birth microbiome, the microbiome you carry in your fifties and sixties is substantially the product of your dietary and lifestyle choices over the preceding decades — and it continues to respond meaningfully to change at any age.

Some researchers have proposed the gut microbiome as a candidate tenth hallmark of ageing — a biological process that is disrupted with age, contributes to age-related disease, and when targeted for intervention, may slow or modify the ageing process. Whether or not that formal classification is ultimately adopted, the practical message is clear: the gut microbiome connects virtually every major system in the body, and cultivating it deliberately is not a niche pursuit. It is a central pillar of the healthspan strategy this book describes.

The dietary changes required to support gut health are not separate from the dietary changes that support cardiovascular health, metabolic health, brain health, and all-cause mortality risk. They are the same changes: more diverse plant foods, more fibre, less ultra-processed food, more fermented foods, less alcohol. The gut microbiome sits at the intersection of all of them, amplifying and mediating their effects. Take care of it deliberately, and it will take care of you.

Chapter Summary

- The gut microbiome is a parallel biological system with over 100 times more genes than the human genome, functioning as an endocrine organ, immune regulator, and neurological communicant. Some researchers now propose it as a tenth hallmark of ageing.

- With age, the microbiome typically shows declining diversity, reduced butyrate-producing bacteria, and increased pro-inflammatory species. Centenarians consistently maintain higher microbial diversity than younger older adults — a signature associated with longevity.

- Short-chain fatty acids (SCFAs) — particularly butyrate — are the microbiome's primary output for systemic health: they maintain gut barrier integrity, reduce systemic inflammation, cross the blood-brain barrier, support neurogenesis, and act as HDAC inhibitors with epigenetic anti-ageing effects.

- Increased intestinal permeability ('leaky gut') allows bacterial LPS into the bloodstream, driving metabolic endotoxaemia — a significant contributor to inflammageing and the development of cardiovascular disease, metabolic dysfunction, and neurodegeneration.

- The gut-brain axis links microbiome composition to cognitive function, mood, and neurodegenerative disease risk. A 2024 Molecular Psychiatry study found that microbiome composition predicted future cognitive decline and depression over a two-year follow-up.

- Approximately 70% of the body's immune tissue resides in the gut. Microbiome dysbiosis drives immunosenescence and inflammageing through reduced SCFA production, weakened gut barrier function, and disrupted immune calibration.

- The most evidence-supported dietary strategy for gut health is high, diverse fibre intake — aiming for 30+ different plant species per week. Fermented foods, Mediterranean dietary patterns, and regular exercise all independently support microbiome diversity.

- Key microbiome disruptors to minimise: unnecessary antibiotics, ultra-processed foods, excessive alcohol, long-term PPIs without clear indication, and chronic unmanaged stress.

References

Badal, V. D., Vaccariello, E. D., Murray, E. R., et al. (2020). The gut microbiome, aging, and longevity: a systematic review. Nutrients, 12(12), 3759. https://pmc.ncbi.nlm.nih.gov/articles/PMC7762384/

Gyriki, D., et al. (2025). Microbiome-based therapeutics towards healthier aging and longevity. Genome Medicine. https://doi.org/10.1186/s13073-025-01493-x

Liang, Y., et al. (2025). From dysbiosis to longevity: a narrative review into the gut microbiome's impact on aging. Journal of Biomedical Science. https://doi.org/10.1186/s12929-025-01179-x

Sonnenburg, J., et al. (2024). The human gut microbiome and aging. Gut Microbiomes. https://doi.org/10.1080/19490976.2024.2359677

Mancabelli, L., et al. (2024). Longevity-associated gut microbial signatures. Gut Microbes. [Analysis of 1,156 fecal samples from 8 longevity cohorts].

Loh, J. S., et al. (2024). Microbiota–gut–brain axis and its therapeutic applications in neurodegenerative diseases. Signal Transduction and Targeted Therapy, 9(1), 37. https://doi.org/10.1038/s41392-024-01743-1

Park, J., & Gao, Y. (2024). Gut-brain axis and neurodegeneration: mechanisms and therapeutic potentials. Frontiers in Neuroscience, 18, 1481390.

Bhattacharya, T., et al. (2024). Gut microbiome predicts cognitive function and depressive symptoms in late life. Molecular Psychiatry, 29, 3064–3075. https://doi.org/10.1038/s41380-024-02551-3

Fragiadakis, G. K., et al. (2021). Gut-microbiota-targeted diets modulate human immune status. Cell, 184(16), 4137–4153. [Fermented food RCT, Stanford].

Wang, Z., et al. (2024). Short-chain fatty acids: bridges between diet, gut microbiota, and health. Journal of Gastroenterology and Hepatology, 39(6), 1037–1046.

Chapter Eleven

Metabolic Health

The silent driver of virtually every major age-related disease — and why it starts years before anyone notices

In clinical practice, I see a pattern that repeats itself with uncomfortable regularity. A person in their mid-fifties comes in for a routine check-up. Their fasting glucose is 5.8 mmol/L — within the normal range. Their cholesterol is borderline. Their blood pressure is slightly elevated. Their waist circumference is higher than it should be. Each individual result sits just inside what the pathology report flags as normal, so nothing is actioned. The patient is told things look fine and is sent home.

What those results are actually showing, taken together, is a metabolic system under significant stress. The slightly elevated glucose reflects a pancreas already working harder than it should to keep levels in range. The lipid pattern — particularly if triglycerides are elevated and HDL is low — suggests insulin resistance is already silently distorting the liver's handling of fats. The blood pressure and waist circumference add to a picture that, in aggregate, describes someone five to fifteen years from type 2 diabetes, significant cardiovascular disease risk, and potentially accelerated cognitive decline.

This chapter is about metabolic health — one of the most consequential and most undermanaged dimensions of healthy ageing. It is about understanding what metabolic dysfunction actually means at a biological level, why it matters far beyond blood sugar and diabetes, how to assess it properly, and what can be done to address it. Getting this right is not optional for anyone serious about their healthspan. Metabolic dysfunction is, put simply, one of the most common and most preventable drivers of biological ageing we have.

What Metabolic Health Actually Means

Metabolic health refers to the efficiency and accuracy with which the body processes and distributes energy. At its core, it comes down to how well cells respond to insulin — the hormone that enables glucose to enter cells and be used for fuel or stored appropriately. When this system works correctly, blood glucose, insulin levels, blood pressure, and blood lipids all remain in healthy ranges. When it breaks down, the consequences ripple across virtually every organ system in the body.

Metabolic syndrome is the formal clinical term for the clustering of interrelated metabolic abnormalities that characterise this breakdown. It is diagnosed when three or more of the following five criteria are met: elevated waist circumference (above 102 cm in men, 88 cm in women), elevated triglycerides (above 1.7 mmol/L), low HDL cholesterol (below 1.0 mmol/L in men, 1.3 mmol/L in women), elevated blood pressure (130/85 mmHg or above), and elevated fasting glucose (5.6 mmol/L or above). Globally, metabolic syndrome affects approximately 20 to 25 per cent of adults, with prevalence rising sharply with age — in the US, an estimated 40 per cent of adults over 60 meet the criteria (Qureshi et al., 2024).

But metabolic syndrome, defined by those five criteria, is really just the visible tip of the iceberg. The underlying pathological process — insulin resistance — begins years to decades before any formal diagnostic threshold is crossed. During this silent phase, the body is compensating: the pancreas is producing more and more insulin to overcome the cells' declining responsiveness. Fasting glucose may look normal throughout this period, because the pancreas is working overtime to keep it there. By the time glucose rises into the prediabetes or diabetes range, the process of metabolic damage has typically been underway for a decade or more.

"Insulin resistance begins years before glucose rises. By the time fasting glucose becomes abnormal, the vascular, hepatic, and neurological consequences are already accumulating. Standard testing misses the disease at the stage where intervention is most effective."

The Australian Picture: A Metabolic Crisis in Slow Motion

Australia's metabolic health trajectory is deeply concerning. According to AIHW data, almost 1.2 million Australians were living with type 2 diabetes in 2021 — nearly three times the number from 2000. Around 125 new cases are diagnosed every day. Prevalence rises steeply with age: nearly 1 in 5 Australians aged 75 to 84 has diagnosed diabetes, with actual rates likely higher given the substantial proportion of undiagnosed cases. Type 2 diabetes alone accounts for 128,000 years of healthy life lost annually in Australia and represents $3.4 billion in annual health system expenditure (AIHW, 2024).

These figures capture only the formal end-point of a much larger problem. For every Australian with diagnosed type 2 diabetes, multiple others are living with prediabetes or significant insulin resistance — without a formal diagnosis, without clinical attention, and without the lifestyle interventions that could alter their trajectory. The three leading risk factors driving the type 2 diabetes burden are overweight and obesity, dietary risks, and physical inactivity. All three are modifiable.

Aboriginal and Torres Strait Islander Australians carry a disproportionate metabolic health burden: First Nations adults are nearly three times as likely to have type 2 diabetes as non-Indigenous Australians. This disparity reflects the intersection of genetic susceptibility with the profound disruption of traditional diet and lifestyle, social determinants of health, and structural barriers to prevention and care — a complex picture that demands specific attention beyond individual lifestyle advice.

Why Metabolic Dysfunction Accelerates Ageing

Insulin resistance and metabolic syndrome are not simply metabolic problems — they are whole-body ageing accelerators that operate through multiple mechanisms simultaneously.

Cardiovascular Disease

The cardiovascular consequences of insulin resistance are severe and now well-characterised. Insulin resistance drives endothelial dysfunction — impairment of the cells lining blood vessels — by reducing nitric oxide production, promoting inflammation, and increasing oxidative stress. It promotes atherogenic dyslipidaemia: elevated triglycerides, small dense LDL particles (more damaging than large fluffy LDL), and low HDL. It raises blood pressure through multiple mechanisms. And it predicts cardiovascular events independently of LDL cholesterol — meaning that someone with normal LDL but significant insulin resistance has a cardiovascular risk that standard lipid panels substantially underestimate.

Dementia and Cognitive Decline

The link between metabolic dysfunction and dementia is one of the most important and under-communicated findings in recent medical research. Alzheimer's disease is now sometimes described informally as 'type 3 diabetes' — not because this is a formally accepted diagnostic category, but because the relationship between insulin resistance and neurodegeneration is mechanistically compelling. The brain is an enormously metabolically active organ that depends on efficient glucose utilisation. When peripheral insulin resistance extends to the brain, neurons begin to struggle with energy production, synaptic function deteriorates, and the neuroinflammatory cascade that drives both amyloid and tau pathology accelerates.

A landmark Lancet Healthy Longevity study in 2024, using UK Biobank data from 176,249 participants over age 60, found that metabolic syndrome was significantly associated with incident dementia, with the risk increasing with the number of metabolic syndrome components present — and critically, with the duration of metabolic dysfunction in midlife. The Whitehall II cohort study, following 10,000 participants for 28 years, found that every additional component of metabolic syndrome in midlife independently increased dementia risk, and that this risk was not fully explained by the cardiovascular disease that often accompanies metabolic dysfunction. Insulin resistance appears to damage the brain through pathways that run parallel to — not simply through — cardiovascular disease.

Cancer

Chronic hyperinsulinaemia — the elevated insulin state that characterises insulin resistance — promotes cancer cell growth through multiple mechanisms. Insulin activates the same IGF-1 receptor pathway that drives cellular proliferation. Metabolic dysfunction also promotes chronic inflammation and oxidative stress, both of which accelerate DNA damage and impair the immune surveillance that normally detects and destroys early cancer cells. Several major cancers — including colorectal, breast, endometrial, liver, pancreatic, and kidney cancers — show statistically significant associations with metabolic syndrome and obesity-driven insulin resistance. This does not make metabolic dysfunction a sole cause of cancer, but it makes it a meaningful modifier of cancer risk that sits squarely within the preventive medicine framework.

The Hallmarks of Ageing

Metabolic dysfunction connects to the hallmarks of ageing covered in Chapter One through multiple channels. Chronic hyperglycaemia and its associated oxidative stress accelerate telomere shortening. Insulin signalling directly modulates mTOR and AMPK — the nutrient-sensing pathways that calibrate autophagy, cellular repair, and the pace of biological ageing. Visceral fat, the metabolically active adipose tissue that accumulates with central obesity, is a major source of pro-inflammatory cytokines that drive inflammageing. And the epigenetic consequences of chronic metabolic dysfunction are measurable on DNA methylation clocks — metabolically unhealthy individuals consistently show biological ages years ahead of their chronological ages.

~1.2M Australians living with diagnosed type 2 diabetes in 2021 — nearly 3x the number from 2000 (AIHW)

10-15 yrs typical duration of insulin resistance before fasting glucose becomes abnormal — most of the vascular damage occurs during this silent phase

~40% of adults over 60 in the US meet criteria for metabolic syndrome; Australian rates are comparable

2-3x increased risk of dementia associated with having multiple metabolic syndrome components in midlife, across major longitudinal cohorts

The Testing Gap: Why Standard Assessments Miss the Problem

One of the most practically important insights of this chapter is that standard metabolic testing in primary care systematically fails to detect insulin resistance until it is well advanced. The primary tools used in routine assessment — fasting glucose and HbA1c — reflect what glucose is doing once compensatory mechanisms have been overwhelmed. They are, in the language of the field, late-stage markers.

Consider what happens physiologically. As insulin resistance develops, the pancreas increases insulin output to compensate. Fasting glucose can remain within the normal range for years while fasting insulin is elevated — because the elevated insulin is maintaining the appearance of normal glucose regulation at significant metabolic cost. By the time fasting glucose rises above 5.6 mmol/L and HbA1c crosses 5.7 per cent, the individual has typically had meaningful insulin resistance for a decade or more, and the early vascular, hepatic, and neurological consequences are already accumulating.

A more complete metabolic assessment includes markers that detect this upstream dysfunction before glucose becomes abnormal. The most practical and accessible of these are:

- **Fasting insulin:** The most direct measure of insulin resistance available outside research settings. Fasting insulin levels above 8 to 12 mIU/L in the presence of normal glucose suggest compensatory hyperinsulinaemia and meaningful insulin resistance. This test is not part of standard GP panels but is available on request and is Medicare-rebatable with appropriate clinical indication.

- **HOMA-IR:** Calculated from fasting glucose and fasting insulin (fasting glucose [mmol/L] x fasting insulin [mIU/L] / 22.5), HOMA-IR is a validated surrogate for insulin resistance. A value below 1.0 is optimal; values above 2.0 indicate meaningful insulin resistance; values above 2.9 indicate clinically significant dysfunction.

- **Triglyceride to HDL ratio:** Elevated triglycerides and low HDL is the lipid fingerprint of insulin resistance. The TG/HDL ratio (in mmol/L) is a practical, inexpensive surrogate for insulin resistance — values above 1.0 mmol/L warrant attention, values above 2.0 mmol/L are clearly abnormal. This information is usually already available from a standard lipid panel.

- **Waist circumference:** The most practical anthropometric measure of visceral adiposity — more predictive of metabolic risk than BMI. Measured at the midpoint between the lowest rib and the top of the hip, waist circumference above 94 cm in men and 80 cm in women (Australian guidelines) warrants assessment of metabolic risk factors.

- **Fasting glucose and HbA1c:** Important but insufficient on their own for early detection of insulin resistance. HbA1c in the 5.5 to 5.7 per cent range — still classified as normal — is associated with measurably elevated cardiovascular risk, and should prompt assessment of other metabolic markers rather than reassurance.

The practical message is direct: if you are over 40, have central adiposity, a family history of type 2 diabetes or cardiovascular disease, or any other metabolic risk factors, asking your GP for a full metabolic panel including fasting insulin and a lipid panel (for TG/HDL calculation) is warranted and provides a far more complete picture of your actual metabolic health than fasting glucose and HbA1c alone.

Reversing Metabolic Dysfunction: What the Evidence Supports

The most important message about metabolic health is one of genuine optimism: insulin resistance is highly modifiable. Unlike many aspects of the ageing process, metabolic dysfunction is not an inevitable or irreversible trajectory. With appropriate lifestyle intervention — and in some cases, pharmacological support — meaningful reversal of insulin resistance, metabolic syndrome, and even early type 2 diabetes is achievable at any age.

Exercise: The Most Potent Metabolic Medicine

Of all the lifestyle interventions for metabolic health, exercise has the most robust and best-characterised evidence base. Skeletal muscle is the primary site of glucose disposal — approximately 80 per cent of post-meal glucose uptake occurs in muscle. When muscle contracts, GLUT4 transporters are recruited to the cell surface independently of insulin, allowing glucose to enter muscle cells regardless of insulin signalling. This means exercise improves glucose metabolism through a mechanism that bypasses insulin resistance entirely.

Both aerobic exercise and resistance training improve insulin sensitivity, though through somewhat different mechanisms. Aerobic exercise depletes muscle glycogen stores and increases mitochondrial density, improving the capacity for glucose oxidation.

Resistance training increases muscle mass — the primary reservoir for glucose disposal — and improves insulin signalling pathways within muscle. The combination of both is more effective than either alone. Even a single session of moderate-intensity exercise improves insulin sensitivity for 24 to 48 hours. Regular exercise — 150 or more minutes of moderate-intensity activity per week combined with two or more resistance training sessions — produces sustained improvements in insulin sensitivity, HbA1c, fasting glucose, TG/HDL ratio, blood pressure, and waist circumference.

Dietary Interventions

The dietary strategies for metabolic health converge on reducing the drivers of insulin resistance: excessive refined carbohydrates and added sugars, ultra-processed foods, excess caloric intake, and the dyslipidaemia-promoting dietary patterns that elevate triglycerides and lower HDL.

Carbohydrate quality matters more than carbohydrate quantity for most people. Replacing rapidly absorbed refined carbohydrates (white bread, sugary drinks, pastries, processed cereals) with lower-glycaemic-index whole food carbohydrates (legumes, whole grains, vegetables) reduces post-meal glucose and insulin spikes, improves HbA1c, and lowers TG/HDL ratio. For individuals with significant insulin resistance or established type 2 diabetes, more substantial carbohydrate reduction — including very low carbohydrate dietary approaches — can produce dramatic improvements in glycaemic control, with multiple trials demonstrating diabetes remission rates of 50 per cent or higher with intensive low-carbohydrate dietary intervention.

Weight loss — particularly reduction in visceral fat — is among the most effective metabolic interventions available. A modest 5 to 10 per cent reduction in body weight produces clinically meaningful improvements across all five metabolic syndrome criteria in most individuals. This is not about achieving an ideal body weight or aesthetically defined thinness. It is about reducing the metabolically active visceral fat depot that drives chronic inflammation, atherogenic dyslipidaemia, and insulin resistance.

Sleep

Sleep deprivation is one of the most under-recognised drivers of insulin resistance. Even four days of sleeping five hours per night in otherwise healthy young men produces fasting insulin levels comparable to those seen in much older adults with established metabolic dysfunction. Chronic poor sleep impairs glucose tolerance, elevates cortisol, increases appetite for high-calorie foods, and disrupts the hormonal environment that supports insulin sensitivity. Managing sleep quality, as discussed in Chapter Four, is a genuine metabolic health intervention.

Pharmacological Options

For individuals with established metabolic dysfunction, pharmacological intervention alongside lifestyle change may be warranted. Metformin, the most widely prescribed medication for type 2 diabetes, has an excellent evidence base for improving insulin sensitivity, is well-tolerated, and has shown signals of benefit for longevity-related pathways (AMPK activation, autophagy) beyond its glucose-lowering effects. GLP-1 receptor agonists such as semaglutide, and related agents — have demonstrated substantial weight loss, cardiovascular risk reduction, and emerging evidence for cognitive and renal protection. These medications represent a meaningful advance in metabolic management, though they are most effective when combined with — not substituted for — lifestyle change. The decision to use pharmacological agents should always be made in consultation with your GP or an endocrinologist.

A Metabolic Health Framework: Testing and Action

Marker	Target / Optimal	Concern Range	What to Do
Waist circumference	Men <94 cm, Women <80 cm	Men >102 cm, Women >88 cm	Prioritise resistance training, dietary change, reduce visceral fat
Fasting glucose	<5.0 mmol/L optimal; <5.6 normal	5.6–6.9 = prediabetes; ≥7.0 = diabetes	Request fasting insulin if borderline. Dietary and exercise intervention.
HbA1c	<5.4% optimal; <5.7% normal	5.7–6.4% = prediabetes; ≥6.5% = diabetes	Even 5.5–5.7% warrants metabolic assessment and lifestyle intervention

Marker	Target / Optimal	Concern Range	What to Do
Fasting insulin	<8 mIU/L optimal	8–12 borderline; >12 significant; >20 substantial dysfunction	Request if not routinely tested. Requires fasting blood draw. Calculate HOMA-IR.
TG/HDL ratio (mmol/L)	<0.87 optimal; <1.0 good	>1.5 elevated; >2.0 significant concern	Diet (reduce refined carbs/sugar), exercise, reduce alcohol, lose visceral fat
Blood pressure	<120/80 mmHg	>130/85 warrants attention; >140/90 requires management	Lifestyle first: exercise, salt reduction, weight loss. Medication if persistent.
HOMA-IR (calculated)	<1.0 optimal; <2.0 normal	2.0–2.9 early resistance; >2.9 clinically significant	Combine fasting glucose and fasting insulin. Intensive lifestyle modification.

Metabolic Health Is Healthspan

Of all the chapters in Part Three — the section of this book going deeper into specific physiological systems — metabolic health has perhaps the greatest aggregate impact on healthspan. This is because metabolic dysfunction does not affect a single organ or system in isolation. It simultaneously accelerates cardiovascular disease, drives neurodegeneration, elevates cancer risk, promotes musculoskeletal deterioration, amplifies the biology of stress, and undermines the microbiome, hormonal environment, and sleep quality that support every other dimension of health. It connects to all the hallmarks of ageing. It is upstream of the majority of the leading causes of preventable death and disability in Australia.

The good news — and I want to emphasise this — is that metabolic health is among the most modifiable dimensions of biological ageing available to us. The interventions are not complex, expensive, or experimental. They are the same foundations covered in Part Two of this book: exercise, dietary quality, sleep, and stress management. The metabolic lens simply adds clarity to why those foundations matter so profoundly — and provides the measurable biomarkers that let you track your progress with precision.

If you take one clinical action from this chapter, make it this: next time you see your GP, ask for a full metabolic assessment. Request a fasting lipid panel (for the TG/HDL ratio), fasting glucose, HbA1c, and fasting insulin. Measure your waist circumference. These simple tests, reviewed together, will tell you more about your biological ageing trajectory and your long-term disease risk than almost anything else currently available in standard primary care.

Chapter Summary

- Metabolic health refers to the efficiency of insulin signalling and energy processing. When it fails, the consequences ripple across cardiovascular, neurological, hepatic, and immune systems simultaneously.

- Insulin resistance — the underlying driver of metabolic syndrome and type 2 diabetes — typically begins 10–15 years before fasting glucose becomes abnormal. Standard testing misses this window where intervention is most effective.

- Nearly 1.2 million Australians have diagnosed type 2 diabetes, with 125 new diagnoses daily. Prevalence peaks at nearly 1 in 5 Australians aged 75–84. First Nations Australians are nearly 3x more likely to be affected than non-Indigenous Australians.

- Metabolic dysfunction accelerates biological ageing through multiple pathways: endothelial dysfunction and cardiovascular disease, brain insulin resistance and neurodegeneration, chronic hyperinsulinaemia promoting cancer, and direct activation of pro-inflammatory and pro-ageing molecular cascades.

- A 2024 Lancet Healthy Longevity study (176,249 UK Biobank participants) confirmed metabolic syndrome in midlife independently increases dementia risk, with risk increasing with both the number of components and the duration of exposure.

- Standard metabolic testing (fasting glucose, HbA1c) detects late-stage dysfunction. Early detection requires fasting insulin (for HOMA-IR), TG/HDL ratio, and waist circumference — all practical, inexpensive, and largely available through standard GP pathology.

- Exercise is the most potent metabolic medicine: muscle contraction improves glucose disposal independently of insulin, bypassing insulin resistance. Both aerobic and resistance training are essential, with effects on insulin sensitivity beginning within 24–48 hours of a single session.

- Metabolic dysfunction is reversible. Lifestyle intervention (exercise, dietary carbohydrate quality, visceral fat reduction, sleep) produces measurable improvements across all metabolic syndrome criteria. GLP-1 agonists and metformin are evidence-based pharmacological adjuncts for appropriate patients.

References

Qureshi, D., Collister, J., Allen, N. E., et al. (2024). Association between metabolic syndrome and risk of incident dementia in UK Biobank. Alzheimer's & Dementia, 20, 447–458.

Qureshi, D., Luben, R., Hayat, S., et al. (2024). Role of age and exposure duration in the association between metabolic syndrome and risk of incident dementia: a prospective cohort study. The Lancet Healthy Longevity, 5, 100652.

Sabia, S., et al. (2022). Association of metabolic syndrome with incident dementia: role of number and age at measurement of components in a 28-year follow-up of the Whitehall II cohort study. Diabetes Care, 45(7). https://pmc.ncbi.nlm.nih.gov/articles/PMC9472484/

Australian Institute of Health and Welfare (AIHW). (2024). Diabetes: Australian facts. AIHW, Australian Government. https://www.aihw.gov.au/reports/diabetes/diabetes/

Varió, A., et al. (2025). Insulin resistance at the crossroads of metabolic inflammation, cardiovascular disease, organ failure and cancer. Biomolecules, 15(12), 1745.

Grossmann, M., et al. (2024). Unravelling shared pathways linking metabolic syndrome, mild cognitive impairment, dementia, and sarcopenia. PMC. https://pmc.ncbi.nlm.nih.gov/articles/PMC11943464/

American Diabetes Association. (2024). Standards of Care in Diabetes — 2024. Diabetes Care, 47(Suppl 1), S20. https://diabetesjournals.org/care/article/47/Supplement_1/S20/

Colberg, S. R., et al. (2016). Physical activity/exercise and diabetes: a position statement of the American Diabetes Association. Diabetes Care, 39(11), 2065–2079.

Evert, A. B., et al. (2019). Nutrition therapy for adults with diabetes or prediabetes: a consensus report. Diabetes Care, 42(5), 731–754.

Lean, M. E., et al. (2019). Durability of a primary care-led weight-management intervention for remission of type 2 diabetes: 2-year results of the DiRECT open-label, cluster-randomised trial. The Lancet Diabetes & Endocrinology, 7(5), 344–355.

Chapter Twelve

Testing and Tracking

How to actually measure how you are ageing — and what to do with what you find

One of the most striking shifts in medicine over the past decade is the movement from reactive to proactive health assessment. For most of medical history, testing happened when something went wrong. You developed symptoms, you saw a doctor, tests were ordered to diagnose or rule out a condition, and treatment followed. The system was designed to manage disease, not to prevent it.

The science of healthspan has inverted this model. We now understand that the biological processes driving virtually every age-related disease begin years to decades before clinical symptoms appear. The vascular damage of cardiovascular disease, the insulin resistance underlying type 2 diabetes, the neuroinflammatory cascade preceding cognitive decline, the epigenetic drift accumulating across every cell of the body — these are measurable long before any doctor would diagnose a problem. And what is measurable is, in principle, addressable.

This chapter is about measurement — specifically, the practical toolkit available to anyone who wants to track their biological ageing trajectory with more precision than a standard annual check-up provides. We will cover three broad categories: functional physical tests that anyone can perform or access;

blood-based metabolic and inflammatory biomarkers available through standard pathology; and the emerging field of biological age testing, including epigenetic clocks and proteomic ageing assessments. Throughout, the emphasis is on what is actionable, what is accessible within the Australian health system, and what the evidence actually says — including an honest account of where the science is still developing.

"The goal of testing is not to collect numbers. It is to understand your trajectory — where you are heading, not just where you are — and to give yourself the information needed to change course while you still can."

Functional Physical Tests: Your Body as the Instrument

Before any blood draw or epigenetic analysis, the human body itself provides some of the most powerful and best-validated measures of biological ageing available. Functional physical tests — measures of cardiorespiratory fitness, muscle strength, balance, and mobility — predict mortality and healthspan outcomes with a consistency that matches or exceeds many biochemical markers. They are also mostly free, require no laboratory, and can be tracked serially over time with minimal infrastructure.

VO2 Max: The Gold Standard Longevity Biomarker

VO2 max — the maximum rate at which your body can consume oxygen during maximal effort exercise — is, by a significant margin, the single most powerful modifiable predictor of all-cause mortality currently known. As covered in Chapter Five, studies consistently show that moving from the lowest fitness quintile to even the second-lowest produces larger mortality risk reductions than eliminating smoking, hypertension, or elevated cholesterol. VO2 max declines approximately 10 per cent per decade after age 30 in sedentary individuals, but this decline is highly trainable — it is not an inevitable destiny.

The gold standard measurement is a maximal cardiopulmonary exercise test (CPET) in a clinical or sports physiology setting, where expired gases are analysed during an incremental treadmill or cycle ergometer test to exhaustion. This is available at sports medicine clinics, exercise physiology practices, and some private health facilities around Australia, typically at a cost of $150 to $300. For practical purposes, many GPS-enabled running watches and fitness trackers (Garmin, Apple Watch, Polar) now provide estimated VO2 max values derived from heart rate data during submaximal exercise. While less precise than laboratory measurement, these estimates are sufficiently accurate for tracking trends over time.

Knowing your VO2 max relative to age- and sex-adjusted norms is genuinely useful clinical information. A VO2 max below 17.5 mL/kg/min (5 METs) in older adults is associated with markedly elevated mortality risk. For adults under 60, being in the top two fitness quintiles for your age — rather than just average — is the goal most longevity-focused clinicians now articulate.

Grip Strength: A Surprisingly Powerful Marker

Grip strength measured with a hand dynamometer is one of the most extensively validated biomarkers of biological ageing in the gerontological literature. It is a proxy for overall musculoskeletal health, correlates strongly with lean muscle mass and physical function, and predicts all-cause mortality, cardiovascular events, cognitive decline, and disability risk with remarkable consistency across populations. A meta-analysis of data from over half a million participants found grip strength to be a stronger predictor of cardiovascular mortality than systolic blood pressure.

Clinical thresholds: grip strength below 26 kg in men or 16 kg in women is associated with significantly elevated risk of frailty, disability, and mortality. These thresholds are used in sarcopenia screening guidelines. Hand dynamometers are inexpensive (around $30 to $60 for a basic model) and measurements take under two minutes. Serial measurements every three to six months track the effect of resistance training interventions with meaningful precision.

Balance: The Single-Leg Stand Test

A 2022 study published in the British Journal of Sports Medicine followed 1,702 middle-aged and older adults for a median of seven years and found that the inability to stand on one leg for 10 seconds was associated with an 84 per cent higher risk of death from any cause — independent of age, sex, BMI, and cardiovascular risk factors. The relationship between balance and mortality is mediated through falls risk, neurological health, and the integrity of the proprioceptive systems that deteriorate with ageing.

The test is simple: stand on one foot, with the free foot resting against the standing leg's calf, for 10 seconds. Eyes open. Repeat on both sides. Being unable to complete 10 seconds on either side at any age under 70 warrants attention. Balance degrades with sedentary behaviour, reduced proprioceptive training, and neurological decline — and improves with targeted practice, including yoga, tai chi, and progressive single-leg balance training.

The Sit-to-Stand Test and the Sitting-Rising Test

Two related but distinct tests deserve attention here. The five-times sit-to-stand test (STS) measures how quickly you can rise from a chair and sit back down five times in a row without using your arms. It is a well-validated clinical assessment of lower-limb muscle power, balance, and functional mobility used extensively in geriatric practice. Normative reference values are age-stratified: completing five repetitions in under 12 seconds is generally considered good functional performance for adults in their fifties; times above 15 to 17 seconds signal significant functional decline and elevated falls risk. The STS is straightforward enough to self-assess with a standard chair and a timer. The Sitting-Rising Test (SRT) is a different assessment — measuring the ability to lower yourself to the floor and rise again without using hands, knees, or other support. It was shown in a Brazilian study of 2,002 adults to predict all-cause mortality independently of age, with each unit reduction in SRT score (out of 10) associated with a 21 per cent increase in mortality risk. The test captures flexibility, balance, motor coordination, and muscle-to-weight ratio simultaneously — a surprisingly comprehensive snapshot of physical resilience. Together, the STS and SRT capture complementary dimensions of functional ageing: the STS reflects lower-limb power and functional speed; the SRT reflects whole-body mobility and compositional fitness.

Walking Speed and Gait

Walking speed is one of the most extensively studied functional biomarkers in gerontology. A gait speed of less than 0.8 m/s in older adults is associated with significant frailty, increased falls risk, and elevated mortality. Maintaining a brisk walking pace — ideally above 1.2 to 1.4 m/s — is a proxy for functional cardiovascular and musculoskeletal health. For practical tracking purposes, average walking pace recorded by a smartphone or fitness tracker over regular walks provides a longitudinal reference that takes seconds to check.

> **84%** higher risk of death from any cause in those who cannot balance on one leg for 10 seconds (British Journal of Sports Medicine, 2022, n=1,702)

> **53%** lower all-cause mortality in highest versus lowest VO2 max quintile — larger than the benefit of quitting smoking

> **0.94** Pearson correlation between a 204-protein plasma panel and chronological age — the proteomic ageing clock (Nature Medicine, 2024, n=45,441)

Blood Biomarkers: What to Ask Your GP For

Standard annual blood tests in Australian primary care typically include a full blood count, basic metabolic panel, lipid panel, and sometimes thyroid function — a useful but limited picture. A more comprehensive healthspan-oriented blood panel adds several markers that provide earlier and more sensitive signals of ageing-related pathology. Most of these are Medicare-rebatable with appropriate clinical indication, and none require referral to a specialist.

Metabolic Markers

As covered in detail in Chapter Eleven, the metabolic markers most useful for early detection of insulin resistance and metabolic dysfunction are fasting insulin (for HOMA-IR calculation), the triglyceride to HDL cholesterol ratio (TG/HDL), fasting glucose, and HbA1c. Together, these provide a far more complete picture of metabolic health than glucose and HbA1c alone. For anyone over 40 with any central adiposity or family history of metabolic disease, requesting fasting insulin alongside a standard lipid and metabolic panel is a straightforward and high-value step.

Inflammatory Markers

Chronic low-grade inflammation — inflammageing — is one of the primary biological mechanisms driving accelerated ageing across all organ systems. Two blood markers are particularly useful for tracking inflammatory status:

High-sensitivity C-reactive protein (hs-CRP) is an acute-phase protein produced by the liver in response to systemic inflammation. Concentrations below 1 mg/L are associated with low cardiovascular risk; 1 to 3 mg/L are moderate; above 3 mg/L (in the absence of acute infection or inflammatory condition) indicate elevated chronic inflammation associated with accelerated biological ageing. hs-CRP is typically Medicare-rebatable when cardiovascular risk assessment is indicated. It is a general marker — it does not specify the source of inflammation — but as a longitudinal tracking tool for the effect of lifestyle interventions on systemic inflammation, it is highly practical.

Interleukin-6 (IL-6) is a pro-inflammatory cytokine that more specifically reflects the chronic inflammatory environment associated with inflammageing. It is less commonly measured in routine practice but is available through standard pathology laboratories. Elevated IL-6 is independently predictive of frailty, cognitive decline, and cardiovascular events. For individuals with elevated hs-CRP on standard testing, IL-6 adds useful mechanistic context.

Hormonal and Nutritional Markers

Several hormonal and nutritional markers are worth assessing as part of a healthspan panel, particularly in the context of symptoms or risk factors:

- **Vitamin D (25-hydroxyvitamin D):**
  Deficiency is extraordinarily common in Australia despite abundant sunshine — largely because sun avoidance behaviours for skin cancer prevention have created a widespread deficiency problem at northern latitudes. Optimal levels for immune function, bone health, muscle function, and mood are generally considered to be 75 to 150 nmol/L.

Levels below 50 nmol/L are deficient. Testing is Medicare-rebatable for high-risk individuals.

- **Thyroid function (TSH, free T3, free T4):** Thyroid dysfunction is common with ageing, particularly subclinical hypothyroidism in women over 50, and has significant effects on energy, mood, cognitive function, and metabolic rate. TSH alone is a reasonable screen; adding free T3 and free T4 provides a more complete picture in symptomatic individuals. For those with persistent fatigue or symptoms of hypothyroidism despite 'normal' TSH and free T4, reverse T3 (rT3) is a useful advanced marker. Reverse T3 is an inactive form of T3 produced when the body converts T4 by a different enzymatic pathway — one that increases under physiological stress, caloric restriction, inflammation, or significant illness. Elevated rT3 can competitively block active T3 from binding to thyroid receptors, producing functional hypothyroid symptoms even when standard thyroid markers appear normal. The free T3 to reverse T3 ratio is used by functional medicine practitioners as a more sensitive indicator of tissue-level thyroid function; a ratio below approximately 0.02 (in SI units) is considered functionally low. Reverse T3 testing is available through most major Australian pathology laboratories, typically on private request outside standard Medicare-rebatable panels.

- **Sex hormones:** As covered in Chapter Nine, assessing oestradiol, progesterone, and testosterone (total and free) is warranted in the context of symptoms suggestive of hormonal decline in both men and women. DHEA-S provides additional context on adrenal androgen reserve. These are not universally indicated but should be part of the assessment for anyone experiencing significant changes in energy, body composition, mood, libido, or cognitive function.

- **Apolipoprotein B (ApoB):** Standard lipid panels report LDL cholesterol, which reflects the total cholesterol content of LDL particles. ApoB measures the number of atherogenic lipoprotein particles directly, and is a more accurate predictor of cardiovascular risk — particularly in people with insulin resistance, where LDL cholesterol may be relatively normal but particle number is elevated. Increasingly recommended as a superior cardiovascular risk marker by lipidology guidelines.

- **Ferritin and iron studies:** Iron deficiency is a common and under-recognised cause of fatigue, reduced exercise capacity, and cognitive impairment — particularly in premenopausal women. Elevated ferritin, conversely, is a marker of chronic inflammation and iron overload conditions. Both ends of the spectrum warrant attention in a comprehensive panel.

Biological Age Testing: The Emerging Frontier

Perhaps the most exciting — and most commercially hyped — area of healthspan testing is the direct measurement of biological age: an assessment of how old your body is at a cellular or molecular level, independent of how many years you have been alive. This field is advancing rapidly, and the science is genuinely impressive, though it is important to understand both what these tests can and cannot currently tell you.

Epigenetic Clocks: The Current Gold Standard

DNA methylation — the addition of methyl groups to specific sites on the genome — changes in predictable patterns as we age. Epigenetic clocks are algorithms that use the methylation state of hundreds to thousands of specific genomic sites to estimate biological age. They are the most extensively validated biological age biomarkers available.

The first-generation clocks — Horvath's clock (2013) and the Hannum clock — were trained to predict chronological age from blood methylation data. They are highly accurate at estimating age but are less useful for predicting health outcomes. Second-generation clocks are more valuable for practical healthspan assessment: PhenoAge (Levine et al., 2018) was trained to predict phenotypic age — a composite of nine clinical biomarkers including albumin, glucose, creatinine, CRP, and white cell count — and correlates strongly with mortality, cardiovascular disease risk, and cognitive decline. GrimAge (Lu et al., 2019) was trained to predict lifespan directly and is among the strongest predictors of mortality available in any biological test system. A large comparative study of 14 epigenetic clocks across 18,859 individuals found that second-generation clocks — particularly GrimAge and PhenoAge — substantially outperformed first-generation clocks in predicting disease incidence and mortality.

DunedinPACE (2022) represents a third-generation approach that measures the pace of ageing — how fast someone is currently ageing, rather than their biological age at a single time point. This is conceptually important: it reflects the rate of biological change, making it particularly sensitive to detecting the effects of lifestyle interventions over time.

Epigenetic clock tests are currently available commercially, primarily through direct-to-consumer testing companies operating internationally. Prices vary from around \$300 to \$600 AUD for a comprehensive panel. Sample collection varies by provider: some panels require a blood draw processed at an accredited laboratory (typically shipped overseas), while others accept a saliva sample or buccal (cheek) swab collected at home — making them genuinely accessible without a clinical appointment. The first epigenetic clock was actually validated using saliva samples, and research confirms that well-validated clocks including GrimAge v2 and DunedinPACE show good cross-tissue correspondence when applied to saliva with appropriate cell-composition adjustments. Blood-based testing is generally considered the gold standard for the most predictive second and third-generation clocks, but saliva-based options meaningfully lower the barrier to access. Several Australian longevity medicine practices now offer these tests as part of comprehensive health assessments. It is important to use an accredited laboratory and to interpret results with a clinician familiar with the field — the numbers are meaningless without appropriate context.

The Proteomic Ageing Clock

A landmark study published in Nature Medicine in 2024, using UK Biobank data from 45,441 participants, developed a proteomic ageing clock based on 204 plasma proteins selected from a panel of 2,897. The clock predicted chronological age with a Pearson correlation of 0.94 and was associated with the incidence of 18 major chronic diseases including cardiovascular disease, diabetes, neurodegeneration, and cancer, as well as all-cause mortality. Importantly, it also correlated with physical and cognitive functional measures including frailty index, telomere length, and reaction time. The proteomic approach captures different biological information from DNA methylation clocks and may ultimately be more actionable — proteins are the functional effectors of cellular biology, and abnormal protein expression patterns may be more directly addressable than methylation patterns. Commercial proteomic ageing panels are currently less widely available than epigenetic tests but are beginning to enter the market.

What These Tests Can and Cannot Tell You

Biological age tests are genuinely exciting tools, but several important caveats apply. First, epigenetic clocks have primarily been validated in populations of European ancestry; their accuracy across diverse ethnic populations, including Australia's significant non-Anglo populations, is less well established. PhenoAge has been specifically criticised for underestimating age in some non-European populations.

Second, a single measurement provides a snapshot — not a trajectory. The value of these tests increases substantially when repeated at intervals (typically six to twelve months), allowing assessment of whether the pace of biological ageing is changing in response to interventions. A single result that places your biological age two or three years ahead of chronological age is not, by itself, cause for alarm — the variance around these estimates is significant.

Third, no epigenetic or proteomic clock currently predicts your individual health outcome with high accuracy. These are population-level risk estimates, not individual prophecies. They are best understood as one signal among many — most useful when integrated with functional assessments, metabolic markers, and clinical judgement.

Fourth, the commercial biological age testing market is currently ahead of regulatory frameworks, and test quality varies significantly between providers. If you pursue these tests, look for companies using validated second or third-generation clocks (GrimAge, PhenoAge, DunedinPACE), processed by accredited laboratories, with results interpreted by a clinician rather than delivered as a raw number.

Continuous Glucose Monitoring for Non-Diabetics

Continuous glucose monitors (CGMs) — small sensors worn on the upper arm that measure interstitial glucose every few minutes — were developed for people with diabetes but are now available over-the-counter in Australia. The FDA approved the first non-prescription CGM in the US in March 2024 (Dexcom Stelo), and several options including Abbott's Libre range are accessible without prescription in Australia through pharmacies and online providers.

For people without diabetes, CGM provides real-time biofeedback on how different foods, exercise patterns, sleep quality, and stress affect glucose dynamics throughout the day. Research in non-diabetic users consistently shows that CGM exposure motivates dietary behaviour change, helps identify individual foods that cause unexpectedly large glucose excursions, and provides visceral evidence of how stress and poor sleep directly affect metabolic function.

However, an important limitation requires honest acknowledgement: a 2024 study from Mass General Brigham, published in Diabetes Technology and Therapeutics, analysed CGM data from 972 adults and found that while CGM metrics correlate reliably with HbA1c in people with diabetes, this correlation essentially disappears in people with normal blood sugar. In non-diabetics, short-term glucose fluctuations after meals — which CGM displays prominently — do not meaningfully reflect longer-term glycaemic control as measured by HbA1c. The researchers' conclusion was direct: for people without diabetes, CGM is best understood as a behavioural biofeedback tool, not a substitute for standard metabolic testing.

Used with this understanding, a two to four week period of CGM use can be genuinely educational: seeing your glucose response to a bowl of white rice versus legumes, or watching it spike during a stressful presentation, or observing how it stabilises on nights of good sleep versus poor sleep, builds the kind of embodied understanding that abstract advice rarely achieves. Most experts recommend short, periodic monitoring windows rather than continuous long-term use. Extended monitoring without clear purpose can promote unhealthy preoccupation with glucose numbers without corresponding health benefit.

Building Your Personal Tracking System

The practical challenge with healthspan testing is not a shortage of available tools — it is making sensible choices about which tools to use, at what frequency, and how to integrate the information into meaningful action. More data is not inherently better. Testing that produces anxiety, obsessive monitoring, or decision paralysis is not serving its purpose. The goal is a minimal, high-signal set of measures that genuinely inform the trajectory you are on and the impact of what you are doing to change it.

The following framework organises available tools by accessibility, evidence quality, and practical value:

Test / Marker	What It Measures	Frequency	Access
VO2 max	Cardiorespiratory fitness; strongest modifiable longevity predictor	Annually or when fitness changes	Sports physiology clinic; estimated by fitness trackers
Grip strength	Musculoskeletal health, sarcopenia risk, mortality predictor	Every 3–6 months	Hand dynamometer ($30–60); GP or physio
Single-leg balance	Neurological health, fall risk, functional ageing	Monthly self-test	Self-assessed; free
Waist circumference	Visceral adiposity; metabolic syndrome risk	Monthly	Tape measure; self-assessed
Fasting glucose + HbA1c	Glycaemic control; standard metabolic screen	Annually or 6-monthly if at risk	GP pathology; Medicare-rebatable

Test / Marker	What It Measures	Frequency	Access
Fasting insulin + HOMA-IR	Early insulin resistance; precedes glucose abnormality by years	Annually if metabolic risk factors present	GP pathology; Medicare-rebatable with indication
TG/HDL ratio	Metabolic syndrome marker; insulin resistance surrogate	With standard lipid panel	GP pathology; standard lipid panel
hs-CRP	Systemic inflammation; inflammageing marker	Annually; 3-monthly during intensive intervention	GP pathology; Medicare-rebatable
ApoB	Atherogenic lipoprotein particle count; superior CV risk marker	Annually with lipid panel	GP pathology; occasionally requires private request
Vitamin D (25-OH)	Immune, bone, muscle, mood function	Annually; 3-monthly while correcting deficiency	GP pathology; Medicare-rebatable for at-risk groups
Epigenetic clock (GrimAge / DunedinPACE)	Biological age; pace of ageing	Every 6–12 months if tracking intervention response	Private testing; ~$300–600 AUD; longevity practices
CGM (2–4 week window)	Real-time glucose dynamics; metabolic biofeedback	Periodic (not continuous)	Over-the-counter pharmacy; ~$80–120 per sensor

Functional Pathology: A Deeper Look When Standard Tests Fall Short

Beyond the standard pathology tests available through your GP, a growing toolkit of functional medicine investigations can provide deeper insights into hormonal function, cellular energy metabolism, microbiome health, and nutritional status. These tests tend to be more expensive, require interpretation by clinicians familiar with functional medicine, and sit at varying points on the evidence spectrum. None of them replace the foundational tests discussed earlier in this chapter. But for people with complex or unexplained symptoms — chronic fatigue, hormone-related complaints, gut dysfunction, or a desire to understand their health at a more granular level — they can be genuinely illuminating when used appropriately.

The DUTCH Test: Comprehensive Hormone Metabolite Testing

Standard blood hormone tests — measuring oestradiol, testosterone, progesterone, or cortisol from a single blood draw — give you a snapshot of a hormone level at one moment in time. This is useful, but incomplete. Hormones fluctuate substantially across the day and across the menstrual cycle, and what your body does with a hormone after it is produced — how it metabolises and clears it — matters just as much as the level itself.

The DUTCH test (Dried Urine Test for Comprehensive Hormones), developed by Precision Analytical, addresses this gap. Rather than a single blood measurement, the DUTCH Complete panel analyses dried urine collected across four to five time points over 24 hours, allowing assessment of both hormone levels and their metabolites — the downstream breakdown products that reveal how the body is processing and clearing each hormone. Using liquid chromatography tandem mass spectrometry (LC-MS/MS), the test measures approximately 35 hormones and metabolites including the three forms of oestrogen (oestradiol E2, oestrone E1, oestriol E3), progesterone metabolites, testosterone and its metabolites, DHEA-S, cortisol and cortisone across the diurnal curve, and melatonin. It also includes the cortisol awakening response (CAR) — the spike in cortisol that normally occurs in the first 30 to 60 minutes after waking, which is a particularly sensitive measure of stress axis function and HPA resilience.

The clinical value of the DUTCH test lies particularly in understanding oestrogen metabolism. Oestradiol is metabolised by the liver along several pathways, producing metabolites with very different biological profiles. The 2-hydroxy pathway produces oestrogen metabolites that are relatively protective; the 4-hydroxy pathway produces reactive metabolites that can damage DNA; and the 16-hydroxy pathway produces metabolites associated with oestrogen-sensitive tissue proliferation. A standard blood oestradiol measurement tells you nothing about which pathway is dominant in an individual. The DUTCH test does — and this information has real clinical relevance for women considering or on MHT, those with a personal or family history of breast or endometrial cancer, or anyone with unexplained hormonal symptoms. Similarly, understanding whether low progesterone symptoms reflect low production or rapid clearance, or whether fatigue reflects a flat cortisol curve or a blunted morning cortisol response, requires the kind of dynamic, metabolite-level picture the DUTCH provides.

One important caveat: while the DUTCH test is backed by a growing body of peer-reviewed evidence and is validated using gold-standard analytical methods, the validation studies were largely conducted by Precision Analytical itself rather than independent research groups. It is not an FDA-cleared diagnostic test, and interpretation of results requires a clinician experienced in functional medicine. Used appropriately — as a complement to clinical assessment and standard pathology, not as a replacement — it is one of the most information-rich hormone investigations currently available. In Australia, the DUTCH Complete is available through integrative and functional medicine practitioners at a cost of approximately $350 to $500 AUD. Cycling premenopausal women collect on days 19 to 22 of their cycle; postmenopausal women and men can collect on any day.

EndomAP: Australia's Equivalent of the DUTCH

For Australian practitioners and patients, NutriPATH's EndoMAP (test code 1501) serves as the local equivalent of the DUTCH Complete panel. Like the DUTCH, it uses dried urine samples collected at four time points across the day and employs LC-MS/MS analysis to measure 35 or more hormone markers and metabolites — covering the full oestrogen cascade (E1, E2, E3, and their 2-hydroxy, 4-hydroxy, 16-hydroxy, and methoxy metabolites), progesterone and its metabolites including allopregnanolone, androgens (DHEA, androstenedione, testosterone, DHT and downstream metabolites), cortisol and cortisone diurnal patterns, DHEA-S, and melatonin. The cortisol awakening response is included as a dynamic measure of HPA axis function and stress resilience.

Where the EndoMAP goes further than the DUTCH Complete is in the inclusion of environmental and toxicant markers — a genuinely useful addition given the well-established role of endocrine-disrupting chemicals in hormonal health. The panel includes BPA (bisphenol A), a ubiquitous plastics chemical that mimics oestrogen, and selected heavy metals that can interfere with hormone receptor function, fertility, and metabolic health. This makes the EndoMAP particularly valuable for patients with complex or treatment-resistant hormonal symptoms where environmental drivers may be playing an unrecognised role. Selected organic acid markers — including 8-OHdG (oxidative stress) and B-vitamin functional markers relevant to hormone metabolism — are also included, making it a more comprehensive functional snapshot than a standalone hormone panel. NutriPATH also offers the EndoSTAT (code 1502, the core hormone panel without the organic acid and environmental additions) and the AdrenoSCAN (code 1504, focused specifically on adrenal and stress hormone patterns) for practitioners who want targeted rather than comprehensive assessment.

The EndoMAP kit is sent directly to the patient for home collection with detailed written and video instructions. Cycling premenopausal women collect on days 19 to 22 of their cycle; postmenopausal women and men can collect on any day. The test is available through integrative and functional medicine practitioners across Australia, with NutriPATH operating on a practitioner-referral model; results are intended to be interpreted in consultation with a clinician rather than delivered as a raw report. The approximate cost of the EndoMAP is $300 to $350 AUD for the laboratory analysis. The EndoMAP and DUTCH are clinically equivalent for most purposes — practitioners familiar with either can use both, with test selection typically guided by which laboratory their practice has an established relationship with, or by whether the environmental toxicant markers are clinically relevant for a given patient.

NAD+ Testing: Measuring Your Cellular Energy Currency

NAD+ (nicotinamide adenine dinucleotide) is a coenzyme involved in over 500 cellular processes including energy production via the mitochondrial electron transport chain, DNA repair via PARP enzymes, and cellular longevity signalling via the sirtuin proteins. It is, in effect, one of the most fundamental molecules in cellular biology — and its levels decline substantially with age. By the time most people reach their fifties, whole-blood NAD+ levels have fallen to a fraction of those seen in young adults. This age-related decline is now recognised as a significant contributor to the metabolic and neurological features of biological ageing, and is the scientific rationale behind the rapidly growing market for NAD+ precursor supplements (NMN and NR, discussed in Chapter Thirteen).

Until recently, accurate measurement of NAD+ levels outside a research laboratory was not practically possible. This has changed. Intracellular NAD+ testing using liquid chromatography tandem mass spectrometry (LC-MS/MS) is now available commercially through several providers, including dried blood spot finger-prick tests sent to CLIA-certified laboratories. The test measures NAD+ levels within blood cells — which better reflects intracellular status than plasma, where NAD+ is largely absent — and compares your result against age-matched reference ranges. Published research suggests optimal whole-blood NAD+ levels are approximately 40 to 100 µM, with levels below 30 µM considered deficient and levels below 20 µM severely so.

The clinical utility of NAD+ testing currently sits primarily in the context of supplementation decisions. Because the same dose of NMN or NR can produce very different changes in NAD+ levels in different individuals — depending on age, metabolic health, body composition, and genetic variation in NAD+ metabolism pathways — testing before and after a supplementation protocol is the only way to verify whether a given supplement is actually working. Without testing, you are essentially guessing at both whether you are deficient and whether your intervention is effective. This is the core argument for NAD+ testing: not as a stand-alone diagnostic, but as a tool to guide and validate supplementation strategy. It is most relevant for people actively using or considering NAD+ precursor supplementation, those with significant fatigue or suspected mitochondrial dysfunction, or anyone pursuing a structured longevity protocol where cellular energy optimisation is a priority.

The Organic Acids Test (OAT): A Metabolic Deep-Dive

Organic acids are small molecules produced as byproducts of metabolic processes — the chemical footprints left behind by enzymatic reactions as the body converts food into energy, produces neurotransmitters, repairs DNA, and handles toxins. Measuring their concentrations in a first-morning urine sample provides a remarkably comprehensive picture of what is happening across multiple metabolic pathways simultaneously, from a single non-invasive test.

The Organic Acids Test (OAT), available from laboratories including Great Plains/Mosaic Diagnostics, analyses 76 or more markers across several domains: mitochondrial function (Krebs cycle intermediates that flag energy production bottlenecks); gut microbiome health (markers of bacterial and yeast/fungal overgrowth including Clostridia metabolites and arabinose); neurotransmitter metabolism (markers reflecting dopamine, serotonin, and norepinephrine processing); B vitamin status (functional markers of B6, B12, and folate adequacy that detect functional deficiency even when serum levels appear normal); oxidative stress (8-hydroxy-2-deoxyguanosine, or 8-OHdG, a DNA oxidation marker that directly reflects cellular damage from free radicals); and toxin or mould exposure markers. The DUTCH Complete panel includes a subset of OAT markers — including 8-OHdG and melatonin — so the two tests are complementary rather than duplicative.

The particular strength of the OAT is its ability to detect functional deficiencies — situations where standard serum nutrient tests show normal levels but the metabolic pathways dependent on those nutrients are showing signs of underperformance. For example, a person with a normal serum B12 may still have elevated methylmalonate on OAT, indicating that B12 is not being adequately utilised at the cellular level. A normal serum B6 may coexist with elevated xanthurenate, suggesting a functional B6 deficiency relevant to neurotransmitter production. This distinction between nutrient level and nutrient function is one of functional medicine's key contributions to clinical thinking, and the OAT is one of the tools that makes it practically accessible. It is also well suited for anyone with unexplained fatigue, mood symptoms, or chronic gut issues where standard tests have been unrevealing.

Gut Microbiome Sequencing

The gut microbiome's central role in healthspan was covered in detail in Chapter Ten. Beyond the dietary and lifestyle strategies described there, direct sequencing of your gut microbiome — via a stool sample analysed using shotgun metagenomics or 16S rRNA sequencing — provides a species-level picture of your microbial community composition. This includes diversity scores, the presence and relative abundance of key species (including beneficial producers like Faecalibacterium prausnitzii, Akkermansia muciniphila, and Roseburia intestinalis, and potentially pathogenic taxa), indicators of dysbiosis, and in more advanced panels, functional capacity assessments estimating your microbiome's ability to produce short-chain fatty acids, degrade specific dietary fibres, and influence systemic inflammation. A critical methodological distinction matters here: 16S rRNA sequencing reads a small portion of a single gene to identify bacteria at the genus level but misses fungi, archaea, and parasites, and cannot reliably identify species. Shotgun metagenomics sequences all the DNA in a sample — from every organism present — providing species-level resolution and functional pathway information that 16S simply cannot. For clinical decision-making, shotgun metagenomics is significantly more informative.

In Australia, Microba stands out as the clinically rigorous option. A Brisbane-based company founded by researchers from the University of Queensland, Microba uses ISO15189-accredited laboratories and shotgun metagenomics to identify over 28,000 microbial species from a single stool sample — providing 100 per cent coverage of the Gut Microbiome Reference Catalogue. Their Microbiome Explorer range fuses multiple testing technologies in a single report: metagenomics for species identification and functional pathways, ELISA-based GI health markers (including inflammatory and barrier integrity markers), and RT-PCR pathogen screening. Critically, Microba has validated their reference ranges and biomarker insights against a cohort of healthy adults — the Microba Healthy Reference Model — and backed their 75+ personalised clinical insights by reviewing over 1,500 peer-reviewed studies across more than 7,000 hours of in-house scientific review. This is a level of evidence rigour that exceeds what many standard blood test reference ranges are based on, which are often derived from convenience samples of hospital populations rather than rigorously selected healthy cohorts. Reports include evidence-graded recommendations for diet, lifestyle, probiotics, prebiotics, and supplements matched to the individual's specific microbiome profile, and are supported by one-on-one clinical application specialists for practitioners. The test is ordered through a practitioner, with an at-home sample collection kit sent directly to the patient. The Microbiome Explorer Essentials tier covers the microbiome analysis; the Extended and Comprehensive tiers add GI markers and pathogen screening respectively. Other platforms including Biomesight (uses 16S, consumer-facing) and the Tiny Health platform (paediatric focus) offer accessible entry points, though with less analytical depth than shotgun metagenomics. A detailed microbiome analysis is most clinically valuable for people with unexplained gastrointestinal symptoms, those recovering from significant antibiotic exposure, those on gut-targeted interventions who want to track objective progress, and anyone with significant inflammatory, metabolic, or autoimmune conditions where gut dysbiosis may be a contributing factor. It can also be used proactively — as a baseline assessment of gut ecosystem health — for anyone pursuing a comprehensive healthspan strategy.

A Note on Functional Pathology: Principles for Navigating a Complex Market

The functional pathology space is a mixed landscape. Some tests, like the DUTCH and OAT, are analytically rigorous and genuinely inform clinical decision-making in experienced hands. Others are marketed with claims that substantially exceed the evidence. When evaluating any functional test, the following questions are worth asking: Is the laboratory accredited (CLIA-certified, NATA-accredited in Australia, or equivalent)?

What analytical method is used, and is it validated? Are the reference ranges derived from peer-reviewed research or from the company's proprietary database? Is there published evidence that abnormal results predict meaningful health outcomes? And critically: will the results change what I do, or add to an already overwhelming list of interventions?

These tests are best accessed through integrative or functional medicine practitioners who have been trained in their interpretation and who use them as part of a broader clinical picture rather than as a first-line investigation. They are complementary to — not replacements for — the foundational metabolic and inflammatory markers available through your GP. And like all the testing discussed in this chapter, their value is maximised when they are used to answer a specific clinical question and generate a specific, actionable plan.

A Note on Mindset: Data Without Anxiety

There is an important psychological dimension to healthspan testing that deserves acknowledgement. For some people, tracking health data is clarifying and motivating. For others, it produces anxiety, hypervigilance, and an unhealthy preoccupation with numbers. Neither extreme serves health well. A result that shows you are biologically older than your chronological age is not a diagnosis — it is a prompt. A single abnormal marker in the context of an otherwise healthy picture is not cause for catastrophising. And the relentless pursuit of optimised biomarkers can itself become a source of the chronic stress that accelerates biological ageing.

Use testing to inform and motivate, not to judge or frighten. The most useful frame is longitudinal comparison to yourself over time: are you moving in the right direction? Is your VO2 max improving? Is your inflammatory load declining? Is your insulin sensitivity recovering? These directional signals are more meaningful than any single absolute number. And they require patience — meaningful biological change takes months, not weeks, to register in most biomarkers.

Finally, remember that the tests covered in this chapter are means, not ends. The goal is not a perfect biological age score or an optimal hs-CRP. The goal is the quality and vitality of your actual lived experience: the capacity to do what you love, to remain engaged with the people who matter to you, and to meet the later decades of your life with the energy and resilience they deserve. Testing, at its best, is simply a way of making that goal concrete and trackable.

Chapter Summary

- Proactive testing shifts the frame from disease management to trajectory management — measuring biological processes before symptoms appear, when intervention is most effective.

- Functional physical tests are among the best-validated longevity biomarkers: VO2 max is the single most powerful modifiable predictor of all-cause mortality; grip strength predicts cardiovascular mortality better than blood pressure across large population studies; single-leg balance for 10 seconds predicts mortality independently of standard risk factors (84% higher risk if unable, n=1,702).

- A comprehensive healthspan blood panel extends standard testing to include fasting insulin (for HOMA-IR), TG/HDL ratio, hs-CRP, ApoB, and vitamin D — markers that collectively provide earlier and more sensitive signals than fasting glucose and total cholesterol alone.

- Epigenetic clocks — particularly second-generation tools PhenoAge and GrimAge, and the pace-of-ageing clock DunedinPACE — are the current gold standard for biological age estimation, validated across large population studies for mortality and disease prediction. Results are most meaningful when repeated serially, and should be interpreted with clinical context.

- A 2024 Nature Medicine study (n=45,441) validated a proteomic ageing clock using 204 plasma proteins that predicted the incidence of 18 major chronic diseases and all-cause mortality with a Pearson correlation to age of 0.94 — a powerful emerging technology entering commercial availability.

- CGM use in non-diabetics is best understood as a behavioural biofeedback tool. A 2024 Mass General Brigham study confirmed that CGM metrics do not correlate with HbA1c in people without diabetes — they show real-time glucose dynamics but not longer-term glycaemic control. Short periodic windows (2–4 weeks) are most useful for learning and behaviour change.

- The practical goal is a minimal, high-signal tracking system reviewed annually or 6-monthly, focused on longitudinal direction of travel rather than absolute numbers. Testing should inform and motivate — not produce anxiety or obsessive monitoring.

References

Strasser, B., & Burtscher, M. (2018). Survival of the fittest: VO2max, a key predictor of longevity? Frontiers in Bioscience, 23(8), 1505–1516.

Bohannon, R. W. (2019). Grip strength: An indispensable biomarker for older adults. Clinical Interventions in Aging, 14, 1681–1691.

Araujo, C. G. S., et al. (2022). Ability to sit and rise from the floor as a predictor of all-cause mortality. European Journal of Preventive Cardiology, 29(6), e261–e262.

Araujo, C. G. S., et al. (2022). Standing on one leg for 10 seconds is associated with lower all-cause mortality in middle-aged and older individuals. British Journal of Sports Medicine, 56(17), 975–980.

Levine, M. E., et al. (2018). An epigenetic biomarker of aging for lifespan and healthspan. Aging, 10(4), 573–591.

Lu, A. T., et al. (2019). DNA methylation GrimAge strongly predicts lifespan and healthspan. Aging, 11(2), 303–327.

Belsky, D. W., et al. (2022). DunedinPACE, a DNA methylation biomarker of the pace of aging. eLife, 11, e73420.

Liu, Z., et al. (2024). Proteomic aging clock predicts mortality and risk of common age-related diseases in diverse populations. Nature Medicine, 30, 2450–2460. https://doi.org/10.1038/s41591-024-03164-7

Kusters, C. D. J., & Horvath, S. (2025). Quantification of epigenetic aging in public health. Annual Review of Public Health, 46, 91–110.

Palermo, N. E., et al. (2024). Continuous glucose monitoring metrics and HbA1c in non-diabetic adults. Diabetes Technology and Therapeutics. Mass General Brigham.

Moser, O., et al. (2022). Continuous glucose monitoring in healthy adults: possible applications in health care, wellness, and sports. Sensors, 22(5), 2030.

Chapter Thirteen

Emerging Therapies

What the science actually says about NAD+, senolytics, GLP-1 agonists, rapamycin, peptides, and the frontier of longevity medicine

We are living through a genuinely unusual moment in the history of medicine. For the first time, a serious scientific field — geroscience — is directly targeting the biological mechanisms of ageing itself, rather than treating the diseases that ageing produces one by one. The emerging therapies in this chapter represent some of the most promising candidates to emerge from that effort: compounds and approaches that may not merely manage age-related disease but slow or partially reverse the biological processes that cause it.

This is also a chapter that requires particular honesty. The gap between compelling preclinical evidence and proven human benefit is large in this space, and that gap is littered with promising molecules that worked beautifully in mice but produced mixed or disappointing results in people. The longevity supplement and therapy market is simultaneously generating some genuine scientific advances and a very large amount of commercial hype. Distinguishing the two requires careful attention to the evidence hierarchy — animal studies, small human trials, large randomised controlled trials — and a willingness to sit with uncertainty rather than leaping to confident recommendations.

What follows is an honest, evidence-graded guide to the most clinically relevant emerging therapies — covering what they are, how they work, what the human evidence actually shows, what the risks and unknowns are, and how to think about them in the context of your own healthspan. None of these therapies replace the foundational interventions covered in Part Two of this book. All of them are best discussed with a clinician who understands both their promise and their limitations.

"The most important principle for evaluating emerging longevity therapies: human clinical trial evidence is categorically more informative than animal study evidence, which in turn is more informative than mechanism-only arguments. Always ask which rung of the ladder a given claim is standing on."

NAD+ Precursors: NMN and NR

Nicotinamide adenine dinucleotide (NAD+) is a coenzyme central to energy production, DNA repair, and longevity signalling via the sirtuin proteins. As covered in Chapters Twelve and Thirteen, NAD+ levels decline substantially with age — and there is compelling evidence from animal models that restoring NAD+ levels reverses multiple features of biological ageing. The two main supplemental precursors used to raise NAD+ levels are nicotinamide mononucleotide

(NMN) and nicotinamide riboside (NR), both of which convert to NAD+ in cells via the salvage pathway.

The animal evidence is genuinely impressive. In rodent models, NMN and NR supplementation has been shown to improve muscle function, restore vascular health, reduce neuroinflammation, improve insulin sensitivity, and extend healthy lifespan. These findings sparked enormous commercial interest, and the human supplement market for NMN and NR now generates hundreds of millions of dollars annually.

The human clinical trial evidence is more nuanced. Multiple randomised controlled trials across various doses of NMN (250 mg to 1,200 mg per day) and NR (250 mg to 2,000 mg per day) have consistently demonstrated that oral supplementation reliably raises blood NAD+ levels in humans — that part of the mechanism is validated. What is less consistently established is whether that increase in blood NAD+ translates into meaningful clinical benefits. A 2024 meta-analysis of 12 RCTs examining NMN's effects on metabolic markers found a significant effect on raising blood NAD+ but no significant effects on fasting glucose, lipids, or most other metabolic outcomes. A 2025 systematic review of NMN and NR's effects on skeletal muscle mass and function found positive effects on muscle function markers in some trials but heterogeneous results overall. A May 2024 randomised trial of 250 mg NMN daily in older adults aged 65 to 75 found significantly better 4-metre walking speed and improved sleep quality in the NMN group compared to placebo after 12 weeks. The pattern that emerges from the literature is one of genuine biological activity — NAD+ does go up, and some functional improvements are seen — but effect sizes are modest in most studies, inter-individual variability is substantial, and definitive proof of meaningful healthspan extension in humans remains to be established.

Several practical points are worth noting for those considering NAD+ precursor supplementation. First, individual response to NMN and NR is highly variable, and the same dose can produce very different NAD+ level changes in different people depending on age, metabolic health, gut microbiome composition, and genetic variation in NAD+ metabolism pathways. This is precisely the use case for NAD+ testing (discussed in Chapter Twelve) — measuring before and after supplementation is the only way to verify whether a given product is working for a given individual. Second, not all NMN formulations are equivalent: liposomal formulations have demonstrated significantly higher bioavailability than standard NMN in head-to-head comparisons. Third, exercise is one of the most powerful ways to support NAD+ levels through natural mechanisms — acute exercise boosts NAD+ in peripheral blood cells, and resistance training increases NAMPT (the rate-limiting enzyme in NAD+ biosynthesis) in skeletal muscle. Fourth, nicotinamide itself — a form of vitamin B3 and a product of NAD+ breakdown — inhibits sirtuin activity at high concentrations, which is one reason plain nicotinamide is not considered an ideal NAD+ booster despite raising NAD+ levels.

Safety: NMN and NR appear safe at typical doses used in clinical trials. Common mild side effects include nausea, digestive discomfort, and flushing at higher doses. Long-term safety data beyond 12 to 24 months is not yet available. One theoretical concern — that raising NAD+ could support cancer cell growth, since cancer cells are metabolically hungry — has not been confirmed in clinical trials to date, but this is an area of ongoing research attention. People with active cancer should discuss NAD+ supplementation with their oncologist before proceeding.

> **Consistent** evidence across multiple RCTs that NMN and NR reliably raise blood NAD+ levels in humans — the mechanism is validated
>
> **Variable** clinical benefit outcomes across trials — muscle function and sleep improvements seen in some studies, metabolic benefits inconsistent

Senolytics: Clearing Out Zombie Cells

Cellular senescence — the accumulation of dysfunctional cells that have stopped dividing but refuse to die — is one of the twelve hallmarks of ageing covered in Chapter One and is a significant driver of the chronic inflammation, tissue deterioration, and organ dysfunction that characterise biological ageing. Senescent cells produce a cocktail of inflammatory signals known as the senescence-associated secretory phenotype (SASP), which damages surrounding healthy tissue and accelerates the ageing of nearby cells. Senolytics are compounds that selectively clear senescent cells, and they represent one of the most scientifically exciting areas in all of longevity research.

The preclinical evidence is compelling. Clearing senescent cells in aged mice using genetic or pharmacological approaches extends healthy lifespan, improves physical function, reduces frailty, and ameliorates multiple age-related pathologies simultaneously. The effect sizes in animal models have been among the largest seen for any longevity intervention. The leading drug combination is dasatinib (a cancer drug repurposed as a senolytic) plus quercetin (a flavonoid found in many plants). Fisetin — a flavonoid abundant in strawberries — is another senolytic with strong preclinical support.

Human clinical trials are actively underway but are still at relatively early stages. The most important completed trial is the PEARL (Participatory Evaluation of Aging with Rapamycin for Longevity) trial — wait, that is the rapamycin trial covered in the next section. For senolytics specifically: a 2025 pilot study of dasatinib plus quercetin in older adults at risk of Alzheimer's disease found the combination was feasible and well-tolerated at the doses used (100 mg dasatinib and 1,250 mg quercetin for two consecutive days every two weeks over 12 weeks), with meaningful reductions in senescence biomarkers in peripheral blood. A 2024 longitudinal study examining the effects of dasatinib, quercetin, and fisetin on epigenetic ageing clocks found that while first-generation clocks showed increases in age acceleration (potentially reflecting immune cell redistribution rather than true acceleration), second and third-generation clocks — which are more predictive of health outcomes — showed no significant changes at 6 months. The field is still determining which biomarkers best reflect successful senolytic therapy.

The challenge facing clinical senolytics research is largely commercial. Dasatinib is an old off-patent drug, quercetin and fisetin are natural compounds that cannot be patented, and fisetin is available in health food stores. There is therefore limited financial incentive for pharmaceutical companies to fund the large, expensive clinical trials that would definitively establish efficacy in healthy humans. Most trials are small, investigator-initiated, and funded through philanthropy or public sources. This means the evidence base is advancing more slowly than the underlying biology might warrant. As Dr Chaib, Tchkonia, and Kirkland noted in a landmark 2022 Nature Medicine commentary, the path from preclinical promise to clinical implementation for senolytics requires not just biological evidence but trial infrastructure and funding that the commercial model struggles to provide.

For those considering senolytic approaches now: quercetin and fisetin are available as supplements and have reasonable safety profiles at doses used in clinical trials (500 mg to 1,000 mg of fisetin or quercetin, typically taken in intermittent 'burst' dosing cycles rather than daily). Dasatinib requires a prescription, is not approved for this indication, carries meaningful side effect risk at higher doses (though the intermittent low-dose senolytic protocol appears substantially safer than its cancer chemotherapy dosing), and should only be considered under medical supervision. The honest position for most people reading this book is to watch this space carefully — the next five years of clinical trial results will substantially clarify the human evidence for senolytics.

Rapamycin: mTOR Inhibition and Longevity

Rapamycin — also known as sirolimus — is an antibiotic and immunosuppressant discovered in soil bacteria from Easter Island (Rapa Nui) in the 1970s. It works by inhibiting mTORC1 (the mammalian target of rapamycin complex 1), a master nutrient-sensing kinase that when chronically active promotes cellular growth and protein synthesis but at the cost of reduced autophagy, cellular repair, and longevity signalling. mTOR inhibition is one of the most robust and reproducible life-extension interventions across multiple model organisms, including yeast, worms, flies, and mice. Notably, rapamycin extends mouse lifespan even when started in middle or late life, making it one of the few interventions to demonstrate longevity effects when treatment begins after the biological equivalent of middle age.

The human evidence remains limited and should be interpreted with considerable care. Chronic high-dose rapamycin — as used in transplant medicine and oncology — causes significant immunosuppression, hyperlipidaemia, hyperglycaemia, and other serious side effects. The argument for its use as a longevity therapy rests on the hypothesis that intermittent, low doses (typically 5 to 10 mg weekly, compared to the 1 to 5 mg daily used in transplant medicine) may capture the mTOR inhibition benefits while largely avoiding the immunosuppressive effects.

The PEARL trial (Participatory Evaluation of Aging with Rapamycin for Longevity), published in April 2025, is the most important human trial completed to date. This was a 48-week randomised, double-blind, placebo-controlled trial in 114 healthy adults aged 50 to 85, testing 5 mg and 10 mg compounded rapamycin weekly. The primary outcome — visceral adiposity — did not change significantly. However, women taking 10 mg showed significant improvements in lean tissue mass, and participants taking 5 mg reported improvements in general health and emotional well-being. Adverse events were similar across all groups, suggesting the intermittent low-dose protocol was safe over one year. An important limitation: the compounded rapamycin used had approximately one-third the bioavailability of commercial sirolimus, meaning the actual exposure may have been lower than intended.

A systematic review published in Aging in August 2025, evaluating all available clinical evidence for low-dose rapamycin in healthy adults, concluded that while preclinical evidence is robust, human data have not yet established that rapamycin can extend mean or maximal lifespan or delay the onset of age-related diseases. The authors note that larger, well-designed trials with clinically valid endpoints are urgently needed. The ethical implications of prescribing a drug with immunosuppressive effects — even at low doses — to healthy people who may thereby be at elevated risk of infection or immune compromise remain unresolved.

The honest clinical position on rapamycin for longevity in 2025 is this: the preclinical case is among the strongest in all of longevity pharmacology; the early human safety data from intermittent low-dose protocols is reasonably reassuring; but efficacy in human healthspan extension has not been proven. Some longevity physicians prescribe it off-label to informed patients who understand and accept the uncertainties and risks. It is not suitable for people with active infections, compromised immune function, prior cancer, or those taking medications metabolised by the CYP3A pathway. Anyone considering rapamycin for longevity purposes should do so only under close medical supervision with regular monitoring of immune function, lipid levels, and fasting glucose.

GLP-1 Receptor Agonists: Beyond Weight Loss

GLP-1 receptor agonists — including semaglutide (Ozempic, Wegovy), tirzepatide (Mounjaro), and liraglutide — have transformed the management of type 2 diabetes and obesity over the past decade. But their potential contribution to healthspan may extend far beyond metabolic disease, and this is now one of the most intensively researched areas in all of medicine.

GLP-1 receptors are expressed not only in the pancreas and gut but throughout the body — in the heart, kidneys, brain, and peripheral immune cells. This distribution underpins the increasingly recognised pleiotropic effects of GLP-1 agonists: effects that appear to go well beyond glucose control and weight management. The cardiovascular evidence is now definitive. The SELECT trial demonstrated a 20 per cent relative reduction in major adverse cardiovascular events in people with established cardiovascular disease and obesity. Semaglutide received EU approval as the first GLP-1 specifically for stroke risk reduction in 2025. In the 2025 JAMA Network Open cohort study of over 60,000 adults with type 2 diabetes and obesity, those initiating semaglutide or tirzepatide had a 37 per cent lower risk of dementia, a 19 per cent lower risk of stroke, and a 30 per cent lower risk of all-cause mortality compared to other antidiabetic medications over seven years.

The neurological evidence is generating particularly intense interest. Multiple large observational studies have found 40 to 70 per cent reductions in dementia incidence in GLP-1 agonist users compared to people on other antidiabetic medications. The mechanistic case is compelling: GLP-1 agonists reduce neuroinflammation, inhibit amyloid-beta and tau aggregation in animal models, cross the blood-brain barrier (at low concentrations), and improve cerebral glucose metabolism. A 2024 study of semaglutide in people with type 2 diabetes found a 48 per cent lower dementia risk versus sitagliptin over one year. The highly anticipated EVOKE and EVOKE+ Phase 3 trials enrolled over 3,000 participants with early-stage Alzheimer's disease to test whether semaglutide could slow disease progression. Results presented at the Clinical Trials on Alzheimer's Disease meeting in late 2025 were sobering: semaglutide did not slow progression on the primary endpoint in established Alzheimer's disease. Novo Nordisk cancelled the planned extension. However, researchers have noted that treating established neurodegeneration is categorically harder than preventing it, and the prevention evidence from observational data remains strong. Future trials focusing on earlier intervention — before significant neurodegeneration has occurred — are planned.

The emerging picture of GLP-1 agonists as potential longevity drugs is credible: a Nature Biotechnology commentary in 2025 asked directly whether they are 'the first longevity drugs', noting their anti-inflammatory, weight loss-independent, cardioprotective, potentially neuroprotective, and hepatoprotective effects. For people with type 2 diabetes, obesity, established cardiovascular disease, or significant metabolic dysfunction, the evidence for GLP-1 agonists is now strong enough that 'wait and see' is not the right clinical posture. For healthy, metabolically normal individuals seeking longevity benefit, the evidence is not yet there — the observational associations may partly reflect confounding by indication, and the observational benefits have been most pronounced in people with diabetes and obesity, not in those without metabolic disease.

In Australia, the current PBS position on GLP-1 agonists is evolving but more limited than many people realise. Only two GLP-1 agonists carry PBS listing: semaglutide (Ozempic) and dulaglutide (Trulicity), both subsidised for type 2 diabetes management only. Tirzepatide (Mounjaro), despite TGA approval for both type 2 diabetes and chronic weight management, is not PBS-listed for any indication — the PBAC rejected a PBS listing application on cost-effectiveness grounds in 2024, and it remains available on private prescription only. No GLP-1 agonist is currently PBS-subsidised for obesity or cardiovascular risk reduction, though in November 2025 the PBAC recommended listing semaglutide (Wegovy) for adults with established cardiovascular disease and obesity, contingent on price negotiation with the manufacturer; this had not yet been implemented at the time of writing. For private prescribing of GLP-1s for weight management, Wegovy is the main option at approximately $450 to $500 per month. Saxenda (liraglutide), which was TGA-registered for weight management, was discontinued in Australia by Novo Nordisk from December 2025, superseded by the more effective Wegovy; generic liraglutide products have since received TGA approval but practical access remains limited. The decision to use these medications should always involve a thorough discussion of individual benefits, risks, costs, and alternatives with your GP or an endocrinologist. Key considerations include managing the protein intake needed to preserve lean muscle during significant weight loss (see Chapter Six), monitoring for gastrointestinal side effects (nausea and vomiting are common early in treatment), and appropriate monitoring of kidney function, heart rate, and other markers during ongoing use.

Peptide Therapies: Navigating a Complex Landscape

Peptides are short chains of amino acids — smaller than proteins but with highly specific biological activities as cellular messengers and signalling molecules. Several thousand peptides serve natural roles in the human body, and a growing number are being investigated for therapeutic applications. The term 'peptide therapy' in the longevity and wellness context covers an extremely wide range of compounds with very different evidence bases, regulatory statuses, and risk profiles. It is important to navigate this landscape with care.

GLP-1 Agonists: The Gold Standard

GLP-1 agonists are peptide drugs. They are covered separately above because they have the strongest and most extensive clinical evidence base in this field, with large randomised controlled trials and regulatory approval. They are the benchmark against which other peptide therapies should be measured.

Growth Hormone Secretagogues: Ipamorelin and CJC-1295

Growth hormone secretagogues stimulate the pituitary gland to release growth hormone (GH) in a pulsatile, physiological manner, rather than administering exogenous GH directly. The most commonly used combination in longevity medicine is ipamorelin (a selective ghrelin receptor agonist) combined with CJC-1295 (a long-acting growth hormone-releasing hormone analogue). Together they synergistically increase GH and IGF-1 levels without significantly raising cortisol or prolactin.

The evidence base for this combination in healthy ageing adults is limited to small studies and clinical experience rather than large randomised trials. Ipamorelin was characterised in human subjects in the late 1990s and has shown selective GH stimulation with a favourable side effect profile in those studies. GH secretagogues have demonstrated effects on body composition in clinical populations (particularly tesamorelin, which is FDA-approved for HIV-associated lipodystrophy and has been studied for visceral fat reduction). The principal concern is the theoretical risk of cancer promotion through IGF-1 elevation, given that IGF-1 activates cell growth pathways. The World Anti-Doping Agency prohibits CJC-1295 and ipamorelin as growth-hormone secretagogues, reflecting that they meaningfully alter physiology and carry real biological risk. These peptides should only be used under the supervision of a clinician experienced in their use, with monitoring of IGF-1 levels and prostate-specific antigen in men.

Tissue Repair Peptides: BPC-157, TB4, and TB-500

BPC-157 (Body Protection Compound 157) is a synthetic peptide derived from a protein found in human gastric juice. In animal models, it has shown striking regenerative effects on tendons, ligaments, gut mucosa, and neurological tissue, operating through mechanisms including nitric oxide modulation, angiogenesis via VEGF, and downregulation of pro-inflammatory cytokines. A small case series of intra-articular injections reported symptom improvement in more than 90 per cent of patients with tendon and ligament injuries.

Thymosin beta-4 (TB4) is a naturally occurring 43-amino-acid peptide found in virtually every tissue in the human body, with particularly high concentrations in platelets and wound fluid. It is one of the most abundant and biologically active peptides in mammalian cells, playing a central role in the body's repair cascade: after injury it is released by platelets and macrophages to promote cell migration, stimulate angiogenesis, reduce inflammation, and mobilise stem and progenitor cells to sites of damage. A 2012 review in Expert Opinion on Biological Therapy described TB4 as "a multi-functional regenerative peptide" with demonstrated activity in wound healing, cardiac repair, corneal healing, and neurological recovery. Unlike TB-500, TB4 has a longer clinical research history, including Phase I safety trials in humans showing no serious adverse events at doses up to 1,260 mg over 14 days, and clinical studies examining its use in cardiac repair following myocardial infarction and in dermal wound healing. TB-500 is a different molecule. It is a short 7-amino-acid synthetic fragment (Ac-LKKTETQ) derived from the actin-binding domain of TB4. This much smaller molecule is easier and cheaper to synthesise, is more stable for injection, and can distribute systemically through the body to reach damaged tissues across multiple sites. TB-500 retains some of TB4's tissue-healing properties but lacks the full breadth of TB4's biological activity, which depends on domains not present in the fragment. Most of the available research on TB-500 comes from veterinary medicine and horse racing (where it has been widely used for injury recovery and is now prohibited by WADA), rather than from human clinical trials. The terms TB4 and TB-500 are sometimes used interchangeably in non-clinical contexts, but they are structurally and functionally distinct molecules. For those seeking the more complete biological profile, TB4 is the more thoroughly studied compound; TB-500 offers greater practical accessibility and stability.

The critical honest caveat here, articulated clearly by Dr Eric Topol in a widely cited 2025 analysis of the 'peptide craze', is direct: there are no high-quality, long-term human studies demonstrating improved healthspan or survival for BPC-157, TB-500, or most other non-GLP-1 peptides used in the longevity space. Beyond efficacy concerns, there are safety signals. Animal experiments have found that TB-500 can accelerate dormant tumour growth and disrupt immune responses. BPC-157, by promoting angiogenesis and healing, carries a theoretical cancer risk through the same mechanisms that make it attractive for tissue repair. The FDA has specifically flagged BPC-157 as a compound of safety concern. Neither peptide is approved for human therapeutic use in Australia or the US.

This does not mean these peptides have no future in medicine — the preclinical biology is genuinely interesting and the mechanistic case is plausible. It does mean that using them now, outside rigorous clinical trials, involves accepting a level of uncertainty about long-term risks that should be fully understood before proceeding. An important point of clarity: while BPC-157, TB4, TB-500, and similar peptides are not approved by the TGA (in Australia) or FDA (in the US) for any therapeutic indication, their use is not illegal. They occupy a regulatory grey area: they cannot be sold as medicines or for human therapeutic use without approval, but their possession and use as part of a practitioner-supervised clinical protocol is not a criminal matter in Australia. The distinction matters because patients sometimes assume these compounds are prohibited in the way that controlled drugs are, when the reality is more nuanced — they are unapproved, not banned. What this means practically is that quality control, purity, and appropriate clinical supervision become the patient's primary safeguards rather than regulatory oversight. If you are considering peptide therapies in this space, the non-negotiable minimum is: engage only a licensed clinician with demonstrated expertise and appropriate professional indemnity; ensure peptides come from a TGA-registered 503B-equivalent compounding pharmacy or accredited laboratory with documented purity and quality control; have clear clinical goals and monitoring parameters; and have a candid conversation about the current evidence limitations.

Metformin: The Longevity Drug We Already Have

Metformin, the most widely prescribed medication for type 2 diabetes, has attracted considerable attention as a potential longevity drug — not because it is new or exotic, but because its effects on cellular ageing pathways are unusually well-characterised and its safety record over six decades of use is unmatched by any other candidate.

Metformin activates AMPK (AMP-activated protein kinase), which functions as a cellular energy sensor and master regulator of multiple longevity pathways: it inhibits mTOR, activates autophagy, reduces hepatic glucose production, and activates the sirtuin SIRT1. It also reduces systemic inflammation and appears to reduce cancer risk in diabetic populations across multiple large observational studies. The drug's mechanisms overlap substantially with the biological changes seen in caloric restriction — historically the most reliable longevity intervention in animal models.

The TAME (Targeting Aging with Metformin) trial, led by Dr Nir Barzilai at Albert Einstein College of Medicine, is the first clinical trial designed with a composite ageing-related outcome measure as its endpoint: time to first incidence of any of a cluster of age-related diseases including cardiovascular disease, cancer, and dementia. This trial design has been recognised as a potential model for future longevity drug trials and is currently enrolling 3,000 older adults aged 65 to 79 without diabetes. Results are expected in the late 2020s.

For people who already have type 2 diabetes, prediabetes, or significant insulin resistance, metformin is an evidence-backed component of metabolic management with the additional advantage of potential longevity pathway effects. For metabolically healthy individuals, the picture is more nuanced. There is evidence that metformin may blunt some of the beneficial adaptations to exercise — particularly mitochondrial biogenesis and muscle protein synthesis — when taken immediately before or after training sessions. For highly active individuals, the timing of metformin dosing in relation to exercise may matter. The TAME trial results will substantially inform whether prescribing metformin for longevity purposes in non-diabetic healthy adults is justified.

Emerging Therapies: Evidence Summary

Therapy	Mechanism	Human Evidence	Key Concerns	Recommendation
NMN / NR (NAD+ precursors)	Raises intracellular NAD+; supports energy, DNA repair, sirtuins	Multiple RCTs confirm NAD+ rise; functional benefits variable across trials	Inter-individual variability; long-term cancer data pending	Reasonable if levels tested; use validated formulations
Senolytics (D+Q, Fisetin)	Clear senescent cells; reduce SASP-driven inflammation	Phase 1–2 trials: safe, biomarker changes shown; efficacy trials ongoing	Dasatinib side effects; limited long-term data	Watch trials; Fisetin/Quercetin low-risk supplements; Dasatinib requires Rx
Rapamycin (low-dose intermittent)	mTOR inhibition; activates autophagy and longevity pathways	PEARL trial (n=114): safe over 48wks; lean mass improved in women; no visceral fat change	Immunosuppression; lipids; hyperglycaemia; CYP3A interactions	Off-label only; close medical supervision essential; not for all

Therapy	Mechanism	Human Evidence	Key Concerns	Recommendation
GLP-1 agonists (semaglutide etc)	GLP-1R agonism; metabolic, cardiovascular, anti-inflammatory	Strong RCT evidence for CV, metabolic, weight; observational dementia prevention data compelling; EVOKE AD trial neutral	Nausea; muscle loss; cost; contraindications	Evidence-based for diabetes/CVD/obesity; discuss with GP; ensure adequate protein
Growth hormone secretagogues (Ipamorelin/CJC-1295)	Stimulate pulsatile GH/IGF-1 release	Small studies; no large longevity RCTs	Cancer risk via IGF-1; WADA-prohibited; hormonal disruption	Only under specialist supervision; monitor IGF-1 and PSA
BPC-157 / TB-500	Tissue repair, angiogenesis, anti-inflammatory (animal models)	No large human RCTs; animal data; small case series only	Tumour growth acceleration (TB-500 in animals); FDA safety concern (BPC-157); unregulated supply	Caution; preclinical only; ensure regulated supply; clinician supervision

Therapy	Mechanism	Human Evidence	Key Concerns	Recommendation
Metformin	AMPK activation; mTOR inhibition; anti-inflammatory; mimics caloric restriction	Excellent safety record; TAME trial ongoing; evidence strongest in metabolic disease	May blunt exercise adaptation at high training loads	Reasonable for metabolic disease; TAME results awaited for healthy aging use

How to Think About Emerging Therapies

Navigating the emerging therapies space requires a framework that neither dismisses promising science nor accepts commercial claims at face value. The following principles have guided my own clinical thinking on this subject.

First, the evidence hierarchy is non-negotiable. Mechanism-only arguments are hypothesis generators, not conclusions. Animal studies are informative but notoriously poor translators to human biology — the history of medicine is full of interventions that extended mouse lifespan but did nothing or caused harm in humans. Small human trials are suggestive but not definitive. Large, randomised, controlled trials with clinical outcome endpoints are the minimum standard for confident clinical recommendation. Most of what fills the emerging therapies space sits below that bar. This is not a reason to dismiss it entirely, but it is a reason to hold it lightly.

Second, the lifestyle foundations covered in Part Two of this book are not waiting for validation — they are the validated interventions. Exercise, nutrition, sleep, stress management, and social connection have the strongest and most consistent evidence base for extending both lifespan and healthspan of any interventions currently known. No supplement or therapy in this chapter comes close to matching the mortality benefit of moving from the lowest fitness quintile to the second-lowest (Chapter Five), or the cardiovascular and cognitive benefits of the Mediterranean dietary pattern (Chapter Six). Emerging therapies are most appropriately conceived as additions to — not substitutes for — these foundations.

Third, access to expert guidance matters more in this space than perhaps anywhere else in medicine. The right clinician is not one who is enthusiastically pro-longevity-supplement, nor one who dismisses all emerging research as quackery. It is one who reads the primary literature, understands the mechanistic and clinical evidence separately, can help you assess your individual risk-benefit calculation, and will monitor you carefully if you choose to proceed with any of these interventions. The longevity medicine field has a number of credible, evidence-oriented practitioners in Australia; finding one who operates within this framework is worth the effort.

Fourth, the field is moving fast. The landscape described in this chapter will look meaningfully different in five years. The TAME metformin trial, ongoing senolytic trials, new rapamycin trials, and the EVOKE Alzheimer's follow-up studies will all substantially revise our understanding of what works, for whom, and at what stage of ageing. Staying informed through credible sources — not longevity influencers and supplement company blogs, but peer-reviewed literature, reputable science journalism, and clinician-guided discussion — is the most important ongoing investment you can make in this space.

Chapter Summary

- Emerging longevity therapies sit at varying points on the evidence hierarchy. The critical question for any intervention is always: what does the human clinical trial evidence show, not what do animal studies or mechanism arguments suggest.

- NAD+ precursors (NMN, NR) reliably raise blood NAD+ levels in human RCTs. Functional benefits — particularly muscle function and sleep — have been shown in some trials but are inconsistent. Highly variable individual response makes testing before and after supplementation important. Liposomal NMN formulations show superior bioavailability.

- Senolytics (dasatinib+quercetin, fisetin) have compelling preclinical evidence and early human safety data, but efficacy trials in humans are still early-stage. The commercial model provides little incentive for large trials of unpatentable compounds. Fisetin and quercetin as supplements carry low risk; dasatinib requires a prescription and medical supervision.

- Rapamycin (mTOR inhibitor) has among the most robust preclinical longevity evidence of any compound. The PEARL trial (2025, n=114, 48 weeks) found intermittent low-dose use was safe and improved lean mass and wellbeing in women, but primary outcomes were neutral. Efficacy for human longevity remains unproven; off-label use requires close medical supervision.

- GLP-1 agonists (semaglutide, tirzepatide) are the emerging therapy with the strongest human evidence base. Cardiovascular benefits are proven in large RCTs. Observational data shows 40–70% dementia risk reductions in users vs. controls. The EVOKE Alzheimer's treatment trials were negative, but prevention trials are planned. Evidence-based for diabetes, obesity, and CVD; not yet established for healthy metabolically-normal individuals.

- Growth hormone secretagogues (ipamorelin/CJC-1295) have limited large human trial data. Theoretical cancer risk via IGF-1 elevation is a genuine concern. Use only under specialist supervision with ongoing IGF-1 monitoring.

- BPC-157 and TB-500/TB4 have compelling animal data but limited large human RCTs. TB4 (full 43-amino-acid peptide) has the more extensive clinical research history; TB-500 (7-amino-acid synthetic fragment) has more veterinary/animal data. TB-500 accelerated tumour growth in animal studies; FDA has flagged BPC-157 as a safety concern. Neither is TGA- or FDA-approved for human use, but their use is not illegal in Australia — they are unapproved, not prohibited. Require regulated supply and clinician supervision.

- Metformin activates multiple longevity pathways (AMPK, mTOR, sirtuins) and has an exceptional six-decade safety record. The TAME trial — the first clinical trial powered for ageing as an endpoint — is currently underway with results expected in the late 2020s. May blunt exercise adaptation at high training loads.

- The lifestyle foundations of Part Two — exercise, nutrition, sleep, stress management — have stronger and more consistent evidence than any emerging therapy. They are not optional preamble to longevity medicine; they are longevity medicine.

References

Morifuji, M., et al. (2024). Ingestion of β-nicotinamide mononucleotide increased blood NAD levels, maintained walking speed, and improved sleep quality in older adults in a double-blind randomized, placebo-controlled study. Geroscience, 46(5), 4671–4688.

Zhang, J., Poon, E. T. C., & Wong, S. H. S. (2025). Efficacy of oral nicotinamide mononucleotide supplementation on glucose and lipid metabolism for adults: a systematic review with meta-analysis. Critical Reviews in Food Science and Nutrition, 65(22), 4382–4400.

Prokopidis, K., et al. (2025). The Effect of Nicotinamide Mononucleotide and Riboside on Skeletal Muscle Mass and Function: A Systematic Review and Meta-Analysis. Journal of Cachexia, Sarcopenia and Muscle, 16, e13799.

Lee, E., et al. (2024). Exploring the effects of Dasatinib, Quercetin, and Fisetin on DNA methylation clocks: a longitudinal study on senolytic interventions. Aging (Albany NY), 16(4), 3088–3106.

Chaib, S., Tchkonia, T., & Kirkland, J. L. (2022). Cellular senescence and senolytics: the path to the clinic. Nature Medicine, 28(8), 1556–1568.

Moel, M., et al. (2025). Influence of rapamycin on safety and healthspan metrics after one year: PEARL trial results. Aging (Albany NY), 17(4), 908–936.

Hands, J. M., et al. (2025). What is the clinical evidence to support off-label rapamycin therapy in healthy adults? Aging (Albany NY), 17, 2079–2088.

Lin, H. T., et al. (2025). Neurodegeneration and stroke after semaglutide and tirzepatide in patients with diabetes and obesity. JAMA Network Open, 8(7), e2521016.

Johannsen, S., et al. (2025). Semaglutide in early-stage Alzheimer's disease (EVOKE/EVOKE+). Presented at Clinical Trials on Alzheimer's Disease meeting, San Diego. [Neutral primary endpoint; Novo Nordisk press release Nov 2025].

Sattar, N. et al. (2025). Are GLP-1s the first longevity drugs? Nature Biotechnology. https://doi.org/10.1038/s41587-025-02932-1

Topol, E. (2025). The Peptide Craze. Ground Truths Substack. https://erictopol.substack.com/p/the-peptide-craze

Barzilai, N., et al. (2016). Metformin as a tool to target aging. Cell Metabolism, 23(6), 1060–1065. [TAME trial rationale].

Guarente, L., Sinclair, D. A., & Kroemer, G. (2024). Human trials exploring anti-aging medicines. Cell Metabolism, 36(2), 354–376.

Chapter Fourteen

Finding Your Starting Point

*Knowing where you actually stand
before you decide where you want to
go*

There is a version of this chapter that begins with a checklist. Tick the boxes, add up your score, consult a colour-coded chart. Clean, efficient, satisfying. I am not going to write that chapter.

The reason is simple: you are not a checklist. You are a person with a particular history, a particular biology, particular habits laid down over decades, particular fears and enthusiasms and competing pressures. The process of finding your healthspan starting point is not about slotting yourself into a risk category. It is about developing an accurate, honest picture of where you actually stand — physically, metabolically, functionally, and psychologically — so that the choices you make from here are genuinely grounded in your own reality rather than in generic advice designed for a hypothetical average person who does not exist.

That said, structure is useful. This chapter gives you a framework for taking honest stock of your current situation across the key domains of healthspan. It draws directly on the science covered in the preceding thirteen chapters, and it sets the stage for Chapter Fifteen, which will help you decide which interventions are most likely to move the needle most for you specifically.

> *"The single most important question in healthspan medicine is not 'what should a person my age be doing?' It is 'given who I actually am, what am I currently doing, and where are the gaps?' The answer to that question is never the same for any two people."*

Your Body's Age vs the Calendar's Age

One of the most clarifying shifts in how I think about patients — and how they think about themselves — is moving from chronological age to biological age as the primary frame of reference. Your chronological age is just arithmetic: the number of years since you were born. It is the same for everyone born on the same day, regardless of whether they ran ultramarathons for three decades or barely moved from a desk. Your biological age is something quite different.

Biological age reflects the actual functional state of your tissues, organs, and cells. Two people who are both 52 years old by the calendar can have biological ages that differ by fifteen years or more in either direction. The person whose biological age is 42 has substantially more physiological reserve, lower disease risk, and greater capacity to respond to interventions than the person whose biological age is 62 — even though the calendar says they are identical. This is not a metaphor. Biological age, as measured by validated tools like epigenetic clocks (Chapter Twelve), grip strength norms, VO2 max, and functional mobility tests, is a stronger predictor of mortality and disease incidence than chronological age alone.

The good news embedded in this idea is significant: biological age is modifiable. Unlike your date of birth, it is not fixed. The research we covered in Parts Two and Three of this book describes intervention after intervention that has been shown to move biological age in the right direction — sometimes dramatically, and sometimes in as little as eight to twelve weeks of consistent change. But before you can move it, you need to know where it is. That requires honest self-assessment across multiple domains.

The Five Domains of Healthspan Assessment

Healthspan is not a single thing that can be measured with one number. It is the integrated product of multiple biological and behavioural systems working together. For practical purposes, I find it most useful to organise self-assessment around five interconnected domains. Your picture will be strong in some areas and weaker in others — and that variation is precisely what makes personalisation possible.

Domain 1: Physical Capacity

How well does your body actually work? This domain covers the physical measures that most directly predict mortality and functional independence over the coming decades. The question here is not whether you feel healthy. It is what the objective measures tell you.

The most important single metric is cardiorespiratory fitness, expressed as VO2 max (Chapter Twelve). If you do not have a laboratory-measured VO2 max from a recent maximal exercise test, a reasonable estimate can be obtained from wearable devices or from submaximal field tests. What matters most is not the number itself but which fitness quintile you sit in for your age and sex. The mortality difference between the lowest and second-lowest fitness quintile is larger than the difference between any two medications ever studied in cardiovascular disease. If your estimated VO2 max places you in the bottom fifth of age-matched peers, improving your cardiorespiratory fitness is probably the single highest-leverage action available to you.

Muscle strength and function come next. Grip strength is the most validated and accessible clinical marker of whole-body muscular strength, with reference values by age and sex (Chapter Twelve). The five-times sit-to-stand test is a useful complementary measure of lower-limb power and functional mobility. Beyond formal testing, pay attention to your everyday function: Can you rise from the floor without using your hands? Can you carry heavy shopping bags without difficulty? Can you take stairs without your legs feeling challenged? These functional questions are not trivial — they reflect the same underlying physiological reserve that the formal tests measure.

Balance rounds out the physical domain. The single-leg balance test (standing on one leg, eyes open, for at least 10 seconds) is a deceptively simple screen that predicts mortality risk independently of other physical markers. If you cannot manage 10 seconds on your less dominant leg, this is clinically meaningful information. The Sitting-Rising Test (floor to standing without hand support) captures a different dimension — whole-body mobility, flexibility, and motor coordination — and is worth attempting as a personal baseline.

Domain 2: Metabolic Health

Metabolic health is the domain most likely to have silent problems in people aged 40 to 65. As we covered in Chapter Eleven, insulin resistance — the central driver of metabolic dysfunction — can be substantially advanced before it shows up in standard blood tests. Fasting glucose and HbA1c, the tests most commonly ordered in general practice, typically remain normal until insulin resistance has been building for years.

A more sensitive picture requires looking at fasting insulin alongside fasting glucose to calculate HOMA-IR (Homeostatic Model Assessment of Insulin Resistance), and at the triglyceride-to-HDL ratio, which is a strong proxy for insulin resistance and small dense LDL particle size. Waist circumference (measured at the navel level, not the belt line) is the simplest and most underused clinical marker: in Australian adults, values above 94 cm in men and 80 cm in women signal visceral adiposity and elevated cardiometabolic risk, with risk increasing further above 102 cm and 88 cm respectively.

For a complete metabolic picture, the markers that matter most are: fasting insulin and HOMA-IR; fasting glucose and HbA1c; triglycerides and HDL cholesterol (and the ratio between them); ApoB (a better measure of atherogenic particle burden than LDL-C); and blood pressure — both the number itself and, crucially, how it has trended over time. If you have not had a full metabolic panel including fasting insulin in the past two years, that is the most important blood test gap to close.

Domain 3: Inflammatory and Hormonal Landscape

Chronic low-grade inflammation — what researchers call inflammageing — is one of the most important drivers of accelerated biological ageing. It is also largely invisible without specific testing. High-sensitivity C-reactive protein (hs-CRP) is the most accessible inflammatory marker in routine practice: values above 1.0 mg/L begin to signal elevated background inflammation; above 3.0 mg/L is clinically significant and warrants investigation. IL-6 and other cytokines provide additional information in more detailed assessments.

The hormonal landscape shifts significantly between the ages of 40 and 65 for both men and women, and these shifts interact with almost every other aspect of healthspan. For women, the perimenopause and menopause transition (Chapter Nine) represents a period of profound hormonal change with wide-ranging consequences for cardiovascular health, bone density, body composition, cognitive function, and sleep. For men, the gradual decline of testosterone from the mid-thirties onwards (Chapter Nine) affects muscle mass, mood, motivation, metabolic health, and cardiovascular risk in ways that are often attributed to ageing but may in part be addressed. Thyroid function deserves particular attention: subclinical hypothyroidism is common in women over 50, and both directions of thyroid dysfunction affect energy, weight, cognition, and metabolic rate.

For most people in the 40 to 65 age range, a hormonal baseline should include: TSH (and free T3 and free T4 if symptomatic), total and free testosterone (for men), oestradiol and FSH (for women in or approaching perimenopause), DHEA-S, and vitamin D. If you have not had a hormonal assessment, this is often where the most actionable findings are discovered — not because hormonal optimisation is a magic bullet, but because unrecognised hormonal changes are frequently contributing to symptoms that have been attributed to other causes.

Domain 4: Sleep, Stress, and Psychological Wellbeing

Sleep is not a soft lifestyle variable. It is a hard biological requirement with measurable consequences for every domain of healthspan covered in this book. Chapter Eight made the case in detail: consistently sleeping fewer than seven hours is associated with elevated cardiovascular disease risk, accelerated biological ageing, impaired glucose regulation, increased appetite and weight gain, impaired immune function, and accelerated cognitive decline. Before asking what supplements to take or what exercise protocol to follow, it is worth asking honestly: am I sleeping seven to nine hours of reasonably consolidated sleep on most nights?

The answer, for many people in this age range, is no — and the reasons are often multiple and interacting. Hormonal changes in midlife (particularly for women in perimenopause), stress-related cortisol dysregulation, undiagnosed sleep apnoea, alcohol's disruption of sleep architecture, and chronic sleep debt accumulated over decades of work and family demands all contribute. Sleep apnoea in particular is dramatically underdiagnosed in Australian adults: it is estimated that approximately 80 per cent of people with moderate-to-severe obstructive sleep apnoea are undiagnosed, and the condition has significant consequences for cardiovascular health, metabolic function, and cognitive performance. If you snore regularly, wake unrefreshed, or have a partner who reports breathing pauses during your sleep, this warrants investigation.

Psychological wellbeing and stress management are equally non-negotiable. Chronic psychological stress activates the HPA axis and sympathetic nervous system in ways that drive inflammation, accelerate telomere shortening, impair immune function, and increase cardiovascular risk. The research on social connection covered in Chapter Eight is particularly clear: social isolation carries a mortality risk equivalent to smoking fifteen cigarettes a day. An honest starting-point assessment asks not just about acute stress but about the chronic background level: Do you regularly feel overwhelmed? Do you have people in your life with whom you feel genuinely connected? Do you have practices — however simple — that support psychological recovery?

Domain 5: Nutrition and Gut Health

What you eat, how often you eat, and the health of the gut ecosystem through which you absorb and process everything you consume are foundational to every other domain of healthspan. But the starting-point assessment here is more about patterns than perfection.

The most useful questions are not about specific macronutrient ratios or whether you hit a particular protein gram target on Tuesday. They are: Is your overall dietary pattern predominantly whole foods, or predominantly processed? Do you consistently eat enough protein to support muscle maintenance and repair (Chapter Six: 1.6 to 2.2 grams per kilogram of body weight)? Do you eat a wide diversity of plant foods — the research suggests 30 or more different plant species per week supports gut microbiome diversity? Do you consume alcohol regularly, and if so, at what level? Do you have significant gastrointestinal symptoms — bloating, irregular bowel habits, reflux, abdominal discomfort — that may indicate underlying gut dysfunction?

Gut health, as we covered in Chapter Ten, is increasingly recognised as a systemic influence on inflammation, metabolic function, immune regulation, and even cognitive health. Many people in their forties and fifties have been through significant microbiome disruption — from antibiotic courses, dietary changes, stress, or the accumulated effects of a low-fibre diet — without any clinical investigation of their gut ecosystem. This is not always a priority, but for people with unexplained symptoms, persistent inflammation, or autoimmune conditions, a formal microbiome assessment (Chapter Twelve) can provide genuinely useful clinical information.

Taking Stock: An Honest Self-Assessment

The following questions are not a quiz with a score at the end. They are prompts designed to help you identify the areas where your current reality is furthest from where you would like to be, and where the evidence suggests the greatest opportunity for improvement. Work through them slowly, honestly, and without self-judgement. The purpose is clarity, not criticism.

Physical Capacity

- **Cardiorespiratory fitness:** Do you know your VO2 max or fitness quintile? How do you feel on the stairs, carrying loads, walking briskly for 20 minutes? Would you describe yourself as genuinely fit, moderately fit, or unfit for your age?

- **Muscle strength and mass:** Have you noticed changes in your strength or body composition over the past five years? Can you rise from the floor without hands? Do you regularly do resistance training?

- **Balance and mobility:** Can you stand on one leg for 10 seconds comfortably? Do you have stiffness, limited range of movement, or chronic joint pain that limits your activity?

- **Functional independence:** Is there anything you used to do physically that you can no longer do? Any activities you have stopped not from lack of interest but from lack of capacity?

Metabolic Health

- **Blood markers:** When did you last have a full metabolic panel including fasting insulin, HOMA-IR, and ApoB? Do you know your HbA1c, fasting glucose, and triglyceride-to-HDL ratio?

- **Waist circumference:** Have you measured yours recently? Does it fall within healthy ranges for your sex, or above clinical risk thresholds?

- **Energy and weight:** Have you gained significant weight around the abdomen in the past decade? Do you experience significant post-meal energy crashes? Do you feel chronically fatigued in ways that are not explained by sleep alone?

- **Blood pressure:** Do you know your typical blood pressure? Has it been trending upward over recent years?

Inflammatory and Hormonal Landscape

- **Inflammation markers:** Do you know your hs-CRP? Do you have chronic pain, persistent fatigue, or autoimmune conditions that may reflect elevated background inflammation?

- **Hormonal status:** For women: where are you in the perimenopause transition? Do you experience symptoms — hot flushes, sleep disruption, mood changes, cognitive fogginess — that may reflect declining oestrogen? For men: do you experience low energy, reduced motivation, declining libido, or difficulty maintaining muscle mass that may relate to testosterone decline?

- **Thyroid:** Have you had a full thyroid panel recently? Do you experience unexplained weight gain, cold intolerance, fatigue, hair thinning, or cognitive sluggishness?

- **Vitamin D:** Do you know your 25-OH vitamin D level? This single deficiency affects bone health, immune function, cancer risk, and metabolic health.

Sleep, Stress, and Psychological Wellbeing

- **Sleep quantity and quality:** Are you consistently getting seven to nine hours? Do you wake feeling rested? Do you snore, or has a partner observed breathing pauses? Do you have significant insomnia — difficulty falling asleep, staying asleep, or early morning waking?

- **Chronic stress:** Do you feel chronically overwhelmed? Do you have effective strategies for psychological recovery and stress management?

- **Social connection:** Do you have people in your life with whom you feel genuinely close and known? Have you been more isolated than you would like in recent years?

- **Psychological health:** Do you have persistent low mood, anxiety, or loss of enjoyment in activities that were previously meaningful? These are not inevitable features of ageing; they are remediable conditions worth addressing directly.

Nutrition and Gut Health

- **Dietary pattern:** Is your typical diet predominantly whole foods, or predominantly processed? Are you consistently eating enough protein?

- **Plant diversity:** Do you eat a wide variety of vegetables, fruits, legumes, wholegrains, nuts, and seeds? Or does your diet cycle through a narrow range of the same foods?

- **Alcohol:** If you drink, at what level? Has this increased in recent years? Do you use alcohol as a primary stress management tool?

- **Gut symptoms:** Do you have persistent digestive symptoms that have not been investigated? Has your bowel function changed significantly in recent years?

Identifying Your Priority Gaps

After working through those questions, most people can identify two or three domains where their current situation is furthest from ideal, and where there is a meaningful evidence base for improvement. These are your priority gaps — the areas where focused attention is likely to produce the greatest gains.

A few principles guide which gaps to prioritise.

The first is magnitude of impact. The gap between being sedentary and moderately active produces a larger mortality benefit than the gap between moderately active and very active. The gap between a processed-food-dominated diet and a predominantly whole-food diet produces a larger metabolic benefit than fine-tuning macronutrient ratios within an already-reasonable diet. Consistently sleeping six hours instead of seven and a half carries a larger health cost than the difference between several specific supplements. Start with the interventions that move the biggest levers.

The second is personal leverage. Which gaps are you most ready and motivated to address? Change requires sustained effort, and motivation matters enormously for sustainability. The theoretically optimal intervention you will not maintain is less valuable than the good-enough intervention you will. This is not an excuse to avoid necessary hard work — it is a recognition that the best starting point is often the one that builds momentum and confidence, not the one that sounds most impressive.

The third is interconnection. Some gaps, when addressed, improve multiple domains simultaneously. Improving sleep quality typically improves metabolic markers, reduces inflammatory markers, improves mood, and supports exercise capacity. Regular resistance training improves muscle mass, insulin sensitivity, bone density, hormonal profile, and psychological wellbeing. Starting here produces compound returns across domains.

The fourth is medical urgency. Some findings demand prompt clinical attention rather than lifestyle experimentation: blood pressure consistently above 140/90, fasting glucose above 7.0 mmol/L, haemoglobin A1c above 6.5 per cent, hs-CRP above 10 mg/L (which warrants investigation for acute causes), unexplained weight loss, or any new and unexplained symptoms. These are conversations to have with your GP before beginning an ambitious lifestyle programme — not because lifestyle change is dangerous, but because an accurate medical picture is an essential part of a safe and effective starting point.

> **80%** of the health gains available from healthspan optimisation come from addressing the foundational five: exercise, nutrition, sleep, stress, and social connection — not from supplements or emerging therapies

The Role of Testing in Finding Your Starting Point

Chapter Twelve covered the landscape of testing and tracking in detail. The question for this chapter is more focused: which tests are genuinely useful for establishing your starting point, and which are premature, unnecessary, or best deferred?

The tests I consider genuinely foundational — the ones that provide the most clinically useful information relative to their cost and accessibility — fall into a fairly short list. Most can be organised through your GP, and many are Medicare-rebatable with appropriate clinical indication.

Core Blood Panel

Fasting insulin and HOMA-IR; fasting glucose and HbA1c; full lipid panel including triglycerides and HDL (and calculate the TG/HDL ratio); ApoB; hs-CRP; full blood count; comprehensive metabolic panel (kidney and liver function); thyroid panel (at minimum TSH, with free T3 and free T4 added if symptomatic); vitamin D (25-OH); ferritin and iron studies if fatigue is a feature; and, for women approaching or in perimenopause, oestradiol and FSH. For men, total and free testosterone with SHBG. DHEA-S is worth including for both sexes as a marker of adrenal reserve that declines with age.

Functional Physical Tests

VO2 max (laboratory CPET if accessible, wearable estimate as a minimum); grip strength (dynamometer or approximated by clinical assessment); five-times sit-to-stand timed test; single-leg balance time; and the Sitting-Rising Test as a baseline mobility screen. Walking speed over four metres is a simple and underutilised predictor of functional ageing. None of these require specialist referral.

Cardiovascular Baseline

Blood pressure (ideally measured in the morning before medication, on three separate occasions and averaged); resting heart rate and heart rate variability if you use a wearable; and a resting ECG if you are over 45 and have not had one recently. For those with a family history of early cardiovascular disease, or with multiple cardiovascular risk factors, a calcium score CT (coronary artery calcium scoring) is a one-off, low-radiation test that provides a direct measure of subclinical atherosclerosis and is one of the most useful risk stratification tools available outside of formal cardiac investigation. Discuss this with your GP.

Optional but Informative

Depending on your symptoms, risk profile, and budget, additional tests that provide genuinely useful information include: a DEXA scan for body composition and bone density (particularly for women over 50 and men over 60, or anyone with a history of significant weight loss or high corticosteroid use); a DUTCH test or full hormone panel if you have symptoms of hormonal dysfunction beyond what standard tests reveal; a gut microbiome assessment (Microba) if you have significant digestive symptoms or inflammatory conditions; and an epigenetic biological age assessment if you want a direct measure of your biological age as a baseline from which to track the effects of interventions.

What is not necessary at the starting point: complex panels of obscure inflammatory cytokines, genetic testing for common SNPs (which rarely changes management at this stage), or extensive functional medicine test batteries that generate data without clear clinical implications. The goal of initial testing is to identify significant actionable findings, not to collect comprehensive data for its own sake.

Putting It Together: Your Starting Point Summary

Once you have worked through the self-assessment questions and reviewed your available test results, the goal is to articulate a clear and honest summary of where you stand. This does not need to be a formal document — though writing it down in some form is genuinely useful, because it creates a baseline against which future progress can be measured. It might include:

- **Your current functional capacity:** VO2 max quintile, strength relative to age-norms, balance performance. Honest, without inflation or deflation.

- **Your metabolic status:** The key markers — HOMA-IR, ApoB, TG/HDL ratio, waist circumference — and what they suggest about your current metabolic health trajectory.

- **Your hormonal and inflammatory landscape:** Any significant findings from thyroid, sex hormones, vitamin D, or hs-CRP that may be contributing to current symptoms or future risk.

- **Your sleep and stress picture:** An honest accounting of your sleep quality and quantity, and your current psychological burden and resources.

- **Your nutritional patterns:** The broad pattern, not the detail. Is it working? What are the obvious gaps?

- **Your top two or three priority gaps:** Based on the above, the areas where the evidence suggests the greatest opportunity for meaningful improvement.

This summary becomes the foundation for Chapter Fifteen, which covers how to build your personal healthspan stack — the specific, prioritised combination of interventions most likely to move the needle for your particular starting point.

One final thought before we move on. The process of taking honest stock of your health can be confronting.

You may find that your physical capacity has declined more than you realised, or that your metabolic markers are moving in a direction you did not expect, or that the sleep you thought was adequate is in fact insufficient. These discoveries are not reasons for distress. They are the reason you picked up this book. The research is unambiguous that the human body retains remarkable adaptive capacity well into the sixth, seventh, and eighth decades. Decline is not destiny. But addressing it requires first seeing it clearly, without flinching.

"Finding your starting point is not a clinical exercise in self-criticism. It is an act of respect for the body you have, the life you want, and the time you have to work with. That is enough of a reason to begin."

Chapter Summary

- Biological age — the functional state of your tissues and organs — is a stronger predictor of healthspan outcomes than chronological age, and, unlike your date of birth, it is modifiable. Before deciding what to change, you need to know where you actually stand.

- Healthspan assessment is most usefully organised across five interconnected domains: physical capacity, metabolic health, inflammatory and hormonal landscape, sleep and psychological wellbeing, and nutrition and gut health.

- The most important physical measures are VO2 max quintile (single strongest predictor of mortality), grip strength, lower-limb function (five-times sit-to-stand), balance (single-leg balance), and whole-body mobility (Sitting-Rising Test). These require no laboratory.

- The most important metabolic markers are fasting insulin and HOMA-IR, ApoB, the triglyceride-to-HDL ratio, waist circumference, and blood pressure. Standard annual blood tests in Australian general practice typically miss the most sensitive early markers of insulin resistance.

- Hormonal assessment should include thyroid function, sex hormones (testosterone for men, oestradiol and FSH for women approaching perimenopause), DHEA-S, and vitamin D. Hormonal changes in the 40 to 65 age range frequently contribute to symptoms that are otherwise attributed to ageing.

- Sleep quality, chronic psychological stress, and social connection are not peripheral to healthspan — they are central. Sleep apnoea is dramatically underdiagnosed in Australian adults and has major consequences for cardiovascular, metabolic, and cognitive health.

- Priority gaps — the areas where your starting point is furthest from optimal and where evidence supports meaningful improvement — should be identified based on: magnitude of impact, personal readiness and motivation, interconnection across domains, and medical urgency.

- The foundational tests for establishing a starting point are a core blood panel (including fasting insulin, ApoB, and hs-CRP), functional physical tests, and a cardiovascular baseline. Advanced testing is most useful for people with specific symptoms or risk profiles, not as a routine starting point for everyone.

- Some findings warrant prompt clinical attention before embarking on a lifestyle programme: significantly elevated blood pressure, fasting glucose above 7.0 mmol/L, HbA1c above 6.5 per cent, or any new unexplained symptoms. These are conversations to have with your GP.

- The purpose of finding your starting point is clarity and direction, not self-criticism. The research consistently shows that meaningful healthspan improvement is achievable at any starting point, and that the body retains significant adaptive capacity well into later decades.

Healthspan Starting Point: Quick Reference

Domain	Key Questions	Core Tests	Red Flags
Physical Capacity	VO2 max quintile? Strength relative to norms? Balance and mobility?	VO2 max estimate; grip strength; 5x sit-to-stand; single-leg balance	Bottom fitness quintile; cannot complete SRT; grip strength below threshold
Metabolic Health	Waist circumferenc e? Fasting insulin? Energy after meals? Abdominal weight gain?	Fasting insulin, HOMA-IR, ApoB, TG/HDL, HbA1c, blood pressure	Fasting glucose >7.0; HbA1c >6.5%; BP consistently >140/90; waist >102cm (M) / >88cm (F)

Domain	Key Questions	Core Tests	Red Flags
Hormonal & Inflammatory	Thyroid symptoms? Hormonal transition symptoms? Chronic pain or fatigue?	TSH, free T3/T4, testosterone (M), oestradiol/FSH (F), DHEA-S, Vitamin D, hs-CRP	hs-CRP >3.0 mg/L; vitamin D <50 nmol/L; symptomatic hormonal deficiency
Sleep & Stress	Consistent 7-9 hours? Rested on waking? Snoring or breathing pauses? Chronic overwhelm?	Self-report sleep diary; Epworth Sleepiness Scale; consider sleep study if snoring	Probable sleep apnoea; consistently <6 hours; chronic severe psychological stress
Nutrition & Gut	Predominantly whole foods? Adequate protein? Plant diversity? Gut symptoms?	Dietary pattern review; gut microbiome testing if symptomatic	Persistent GI symptoms unexplained; very low protein intake; majority of diet from processed foods

Chapter Fifteen

Building Your Healthspan Stack

How to assemble a personalised, prioritised plan from everything this book has covered

The word 'stack' comes from the technology world, where it describes the combination of tools and systems that work together to build something. It is borrowed here deliberately. Your healthspan stack is not a single magic intervention — it is the combination of practices, habits, and where appropriate, clinical tools, that work together to produce a biological environment in which you age well. Like any stack, the foundation matters more than the top layers. Add in the wrong order and the whole structure becomes unstable.

This chapter translates everything covered in the preceding fourteen chapters into a practical, personalised framework for action. It is not a prescription — your GP and any relevant specialists are the right people to issue those. It is a framework for thinking clearly about which interventions belong in your stack, in what order to prioritise them, and how to build sustainably rather than trying to change everything at once and changing nothing for long.

The chapter is organised around a simple but important distinction: the foundations, which are non-negotiable and evidence-based for almost everyone;

the targeted additions, which are personalised based on your specific starting point from Chapter Fourteen; and the advanced layer, which includes the clinical tools and emerging therapies from Part Three that belong in some stacks but not others. Getting this order right — foundations first, always — is the most important thing this chapter has to say.

> *"The most common mistake in healthspan optimisation is adding complexity before earning it. Every hour spent chasing a peripheral supplement is an hour not spent sleeping, exercising, or preparing whole food. The foundations are not the boring part while you wait for the interesting interventions. They are the intervention."*

Layer One: The Non-Negotiable Foundations

Five interventions have an evidence base so strong, so consistent, and so broad in their effects that they belong in every healthspan stack, regardless of starting point. These are not placeholders while you wait for a more sophisticated personalised plan. They are the plan, for most people, most of the time. The research is unambiguous: these five together account for the majority of the modifiable health gains available over the next decade of your life.

1. Exercise: The Most Powerful Drug We Have

If exercise were a pill, it would be the most prescribed medication in history. Nothing in the evidence base for healthspan comes close to regular physical activity for breadth and magnitude of benefit. It reduces all-cause mortality, cardiovascular mortality, and cancer mortality. It improves insulin sensitivity, body composition, bone density, immune function, cognitive performance, mood, and sleep quality. It slows biological ageing at the epigenetic level. It is one of the most effective treatments for depression and anxiety. And the dose-response curve means that even modest amounts of activity, for people who currently do little, produce dramatic gains.

Your exercise stack has three required components, each serving a distinct biological purpose. They are not interchangeable.

Cardiorespiratory training — the sustained aerobic activity that drives VO2 max improvement — is the primary lever for mortality reduction and cardiovascular protection. The target is at minimum 150 minutes per week of moderate-intensity aerobic activity, or 75 minutes per week of vigorous-intensity activity, or a combination. But the most important goal, especially if your current VO2 max places you in the lowest fitness quintile, is simply to move up one quintile. The mortality benefit of that shift is larger than any other single lifestyle intervention. Walking briskly, cycling, swimming, dancing, rowing — the modality matters far less than the consistency and progressive effort.

Resistance training is the primary lever for preserving muscle mass and strength, which are critical for metabolic health, insulin sensitivity, bone density, functional independence, and fall prevention as you age. The minimum effective dose is two sessions per week of compound movements (squats, deadlifts, pressing, pulling) at a load that challenges you to near-failure within the last few repetitions. If you are new to resistance training, a qualified exercise physiologist can design a starting program appropriate to your current capacity and any musculoskeletal limitations.

Zone 2 and high-intensity intervals complement the above. Zone 2 training — sustained effort at a conversational intensity, around 60 to 70 per cent of maximum heart rate — is the primary driver of mitochondrial density and metabolic health adaptations, and is ideally accumulated for 150 to 180 minutes per week. High-intensity interval training (HIIT) sessions of 10 to 20 minutes, two to three times per week, are time-efficient drivers of VO2 max improvement and metabolic flexibility. These are enhancements to a solid aerobic and resistance base, not replacements for it.

A practical note on exercise and ageing: the rules change somewhat between your forties and sixties. Recovery takes longer, injury risk is higher if load is added too aggressively, and the value of deliberate mobility and flexibility work — yoga, Pilates, stretching, or simply addressing specific range-of-motion limitations — increases. Prioritising consistency over intensity is wise. An injury that keeps you from training for six weeks costs more in lost adaptation than any short-term intensity gain.

2. Nutrition: Patterns, Not Perfection

The core of a healthspan-supporting diet is not a precisely calculated macronutrient profile or an elimination of specific food groups. It is a pattern — one that has been associated with reduced all-cause mortality, cardiovascular disease, dementia, and cancer across multiple large, long-running population studies. That pattern has the following consistent features.

It is predominantly whole foods. Minimally processed vegetables, fruits, legumes, wholegrains, fish, lean meats, eggs, nuts, seeds, and extra-virgin olive oil form the bulk of intake. Ultra-processed foods — those manufactured with industrial ingredients and additives not found in a domestic kitchen — are minimised or absent. This single shift, from a diet dominated by ultra-processed food to one dominated by whole food, produces improvements in metabolic markers, inflammatory markers, gut microbiome diversity, and body weight that no supplement or drug can replicate.

It contains adequate protein. As covered in Chapter Six, protein requirements in the 40 to 65 age range are higher than previously recommended — approximately 1.2 to 2.0 grams per kilogram of body weight per day, distributed across meals to maximise muscle protein synthesis. This is not a bodybuilder's requirement. It is a longevity requirement, grounded in the critical importance of preserving muscle mass as a determinant of metabolic health, functional capacity, and mortality risk. For a 75-kilogram person, this means roughly 120 to 150 grams of protein daily, which requires deliberate planning but is achievable without supplementation on a whole-food diet.

It emphasises plant diversity. The research on gut microbiome health consistently shows that dietary plant diversity — the number of distinct plant species consumed per week, not just the volume of vegetables — is one of the strongest predictors of a healthy, diverse gut microbiome. The target of 30 different plant species per week, established by the American Gut Project research, sounds demanding until you count: every different vegetable, fruit, legume, grain, nut, seed, and herb counts as a separate plant food. Many people are closer than they think, and those who are not find the goal a useful organising principle for adding variety.

It is appropriately low in added sugars and refined carbohydrates. The metabolic consequences of a chronically high glycaemic load — insulin resistance, dyslipidaemia, hepatic fat accumulation, and accelerated biological ageing — were covered in Chapter Eleven. This does not require eliminating carbohydrates. It requires replacing the refined and ultra-processed varieties with intact, fibre-rich sources that produce a much lower glycaemic response.

Alcohol deserves its own mention. The evidence that any level of alcohol consumption is net beneficial has been substantially revised over the past decade. Current evidence suggests that alcohol is best treated as a toxin that can be enjoyed in small amounts if the other dimensions of your healthspan stack are solid — not as a health food. For people with a family history of certain cancers (particularly breast cancer), elevated liver enzymes, or significant sleep disruption, the case for minimising or eliminating alcohol is stronger still. If you drink, staying below 10 standard drinks per week (the revised Australian guidelines) and avoiding drinking on consecutive nights gives your liver and sleep architecture meaningful recovery time.

3. Sleep: The Non-Negotiable Repair Window

Sleep is not passive. It is the period during which your brain clears metabolic waste via the glymphatic system, your immune system consolidates its responses, tissue repair occurs, hormonal rhythms are set, and memories are consolidated. Consistently shortchanging sleep does not make you more productive. It makes you biologically older, metabolically unhealthier, cognitively slower, and more emotionally reactive — all of which compound over time.

The target is seven to nine hours of reasonably consolidated sleep per night for most adults in this age range. Getting there requires attention to sleep hygiene (covered in Chapter Eight), but for many people the bigger obstacles are structural: work demands, evening screen use, alcohol, and the accumulated sleep debt of decades that makes poor sleep feel normal. The most effective single change for most people is a consistent bedtime and wake time, seven days a week, that allows for the full sleep opportunity without an alarm.

If you have significant insomnia — persistent difficulty falling or staying asleep — the most evidence-supported first-line treatment is Cognitive Behavioural Therapy for Insomnia (CBT-I), not sleep medication. CBT-I is more effective than medication for chronic insomnia in the long term and does not produce rebound insomnia or dependence. Several validated digital CBT-I programmes are available for self-guided use if access to a therapist is limited. Sleep medication has a role in acute and short-term insomnia but is not a long-term solution and some agents — particularly benzodiazepines and Z-drugs — suppress the deep sleep stages most critical for physical and cognitive restoration.

If sleep apnoea is suspected (regular snoring, waking unrefreshed, daytime sleepiness, observed breathing pauses), investigation is urgent. Treatment — whether CPAP, mandibular advancement device, or positional therapy depending on severity — reliably improves not only sleep quality but cardiovascular, metabolic, and cognitive outcomes. It is one of the most underutilised interventions in preventive medicine.

4. Stress Management and Psychological Wellbeing

Chronic psychological stress is not merely uncomfortable. It produces measurable biological changes: elevated cortisol and inflammatory cytokines, suppressed immune function, accelerated telomere shortening, disrupted sleep, impaired insulin sensitivity, and — over extended periods — structural changes in the brain regions governing memory and emotional regulation. Managing stress is not a luxury component of a healthspan programme. It is biological medicine.

The most evidence-supported approaches for chronic stress reduction are: regular aerobic exercise (which is also your Layer One priority), mindfulness-based stress reduction (MBSR) and related meditation practices, structured relaxation practices (progressive muscle relaxation, diaphragmatic breathing, yoga), and — most importantly — addressing the structural sources of stress where that is possible. No breathwork practice can compensate for a chronically overloaded work situation or a relationship that is not working.

Social connection deserves explicit attention here. As covered in Chapter Eight, the mortality effect of social isolation is equivalent to smoking fifteen cigarettes daily. This is not about the quantity of social contact but its quality: the sense of being genuinely known and cared for by other people. For many adults in the 40 to 65 age range, professional and parenting demands have gradually displaced investment in friendship, and the pandemic years accelerated that trend. Rebuilding meaningful social connection is not a soft priority. It is one of the highest-impact interventions available for long-term health.

5. Not Smoking, and Minimising Other Toxic Exposures

If you smoke, stopping is the single highest-leverage healthspan action available to you, producing benefits that no other intervention can match in terms of cardiovascular risk reduction, cancer risk reduction, and respiratory function improvement. The research on smoking cessation support is clear: combined pharmacotherapy (varenicline or nicotine replacement) and behavioural support produces quit rates substantially higher than willpower alone. This is a medical condition, not a character test. Your GP is the right place to start.

Beyond smoking, the most common modifiable toxic exposures for Australians in this age range are excessive alcohol (addressed above), significant occupational chemical exposures (relevant to specific industries), and — increasingly recognised — environmental pollutants including plasticisers (BPA and related compounds), pesticide residues, and air pollution. The practical steps are relatively simple: prioritise organic produce for the 'dirty dozen' highest-pesticide foods, filter your drinking water, avoid heating food in plastic containers, and use low-toxicity household and personal care products where the cost difference is manageable.

> **150 min** minimum cardiorespiratory training per week — the most evidence-supported single target for mortality reduction in the general population
>
> **2 sessions** minimum resistance training per week to preserve muscle mass, bone density, and metabolic health through the decades of greatest risk

Layer Two: Targeted Additions Based on Your Starting Point

Once the foundations are genuinely in place — not planned, not intended, but actually happening consistently — the second layer of your healthspan stack can be built. These are interventions that are evidence-supported and meaningful, but personalised: they belong in some stacks and not others, based on the specific gaps identified in Chapter Fourteen.

If Metabolic Health Is Your Priority Gap

For people with insulin resistance, prediabetes, elevated waist circumference, or a TG/HDL ratio above 3.5, the metabolic layer is the highest priority beyond the foundations. The interventions with the clearest evidence are: reducing refined carbohydrates and added sugars in favour of whole-food carbohydrates;

increasing dietary protein; addressing sedentary time throughout the day (not just exercise sessions — breaking sitting every 45 to 60 minutes with even brief movement meaningfully improves postprandial glucose and insulin); and progressive resistance training, which improves insulin sensitivity through GLUT4 upregulation independent of weight loss.

Time-restricted eating (eating within a consistent 8 to 12 hour window) has a reasonable evidence base for improving metabolic markers in people with insulin resistance, though its benefits appear to be primarily mediated by reduced overall calorie intake rather than the timing itself. Continuous glucose monitoring (CGM) used for two to four weeks provides useful biofeedback on which foods produce significant glycaemic responses for you specifically, and is most valuable as a learning tool at the start of a dietary change rather than as ongoing surveillance.

Clinically, people with confirmed prediabetes or metabolic syndrome should have a conversation with their GP about metformin. As covered in Chapter Thirteen, metformin has an exceptional safety record and activates multiple longevity pathways beyond glucose control. For those with significant metabolic dysfunction, GLP-1 receptor agonists may be appropriate — a conversation that requires full clinical assessment.

If Hormonal Health Is Your Priority Gap

For women in perimenopause or early postmenopause experiencing significant symptoms — vasomotor symptoms, sleep disruption, mood changes, cognitive changes, or genito-urinary symptoms — menopausal hormone therapy (MHT) is the most evidence-supported intervention and should be the first conversation with a GP or gynaecologist who is current on the evidence. As covered in Chapter Nine, the risk profile of properly prescribed MHT — particularly transdermal oestradiol plus micronised progesterone — is far more favourable than the outdated fears from the original WHI trial. Starting within ten years of menopause and before age 60 captures the greatest cardiovascular and cognitive protective benefits.

For men with symptomatic hypogonadism — low testosterone confirmed on at least two morning fasting measurements, with symptoms including fatigue, low libido, reduced muscle mass, mood changes, and cognitive effects — testosterone replacement therapy (TRT) is a reasonable clinical option. Discuss with your GP or a specialist; the decision requires excluding secondary causes of low testosterone and considering individual cardiovascular and prostate risk profile.

Vitamin D deficiency is almost universally worth addressing. Deficiency is common in Australian adults despite the climate, particularly in office workers, people with darker skin, and those over 60 (reduced skin conversion efficiency). Target serum 25-OH vitamin D above 75 nmol/L; supplementation of 1,000 to 2,000 IU daily is typically adequate for maintenance, with higher doses for correction under clinical guidance. Vitamin K2 (MK-7 form, 100 to 200 mcg daily) is a useful co-supplement for those on vitamin D, supporting appropriate calcium metabolism.

Thyroid dysfunction that is confirmed on testing warrants appropriate clinical management — whether conventional thyroid hormone replacement for hypothyroidism, or further investigation and management for other thyroid conditions. Many people with borderline thyroid function and significant symptoms benefit from a discussion with their GP about a supervised trial of low-dose thyroid hormone support.

If Cardiovascular Risk Is Your Priority Gap

For people with elevated ApoB, family history of premature cardiovascular disease, or a significant coronary artery calcium score, cardiovascular risk management is a medical priority that requires partnership with your GP. The lifestyle interventions with the clearest cardiovascular evidence are aerobic exercise, a Mediterranean or DASH dietary pattern, smoking cessation, and blood pressure management. For those with confirmed elevated atherogenic risk, statin therapy — or where statins are not tolerated, alternative lipid-lowering agents — has a strong evidence base that lifestyle alone often cannot match.

Omega-3 fatty acids (EPA and DHA from marine sources, at doses of 2 to 4 grams per day of combined EPA/DHA) have a reasonable evidence base for triglyceride reduction and modest cardiovascular risk reduction in people with elevated triglycerides. The evidence is strongest for prescription-strength EPA (icosapentaenoic acid) formulations in people with elevated triglycerides despite statin therapy, but consumer-grade quality fish oil at meaningful doses provides practical benefit for most people.

If Sleep and Recovery Are Your Priority Gap

For people with confirmed or suspected obstructive sleep apnoea: investigation first. A home sleep study (which can be arranged through your GP) is the appropriate starting point. Treatment is non-negotiable if moderate-to-severe apnoea is confirmed. For people with insomnia without sleep apnoea: CBT-I as first-line, with attention to sleep hygiene practices (consistent schedule, dark and cool sleep environment, reduced evening light exposure, limiting caffeine after noon, and alcohol management). For people with perimenopause-related sleep disruption specifically: MHT is often the most effective intervention and is frequently overlooked in favour of sleep medications.

Magnesium glycinate or magnesium threonate (300 to 400 mg elemental magnesium in the evening) has a reasonable evidence base for improving sleep onset and quality in people with insufficient dietary magnesium intake, which includes a majority of adults eating a Western diet. It is safe, inexpensive, and worth trialling as a starting supplement alongside the behavioural interventions.

If Cognitive Health and Brain Ageing Are Your Priority Gap

The most powerful evidence-based interventions for cognitive longevity are also the foundations: aerobic exercise (particularly zone 2 training, which drives BDNF production and hippocampal neurogenesis), quality sleep (during which the brain's glymphatic waste-clearance system operates), social engagement, and dietary patterns rich in omega-3 fatty acids, polyphenols, and diverse plant foods. There is no supplement that competes with these in terms of evidence or effect size.

Beyond the foundations, the targeted additions with the clearest cognitive evidence include: omega-3 supplementation (EPA and DHA) in people with low dietary fish intake; management of cardiovascular risk factors (which is one of the most powerful modifiable predictors of dementia incidence); treatment of depression and anxiety (which are both risk factors for dementia and treatable conditions); and optimised management of sleep (particularly sleep apnoea, which is strongly associated with accelerated cognitive decline).

For those with a family history of Alzheimer's disease or carrying the APOE4 allele (which approximately 25 per cent of the population carries in at least one copy, and which triples dementia risk in carriers of two copies), more aggressive cardiovascular and metabolic risk management, earlier MHT consideration for women, and careful attention to sleep quality are particularly high priorities. Genetic testing for APOE status is available; the decision to know this information is personal and should be made after appropriate counselling about what the result means and does not mean in terms of clinical management.

If Gut Health Is Your Priority Gap

For people with persistent gastrointestinal symptoms, recurrent infections, autoimmune conditions, or significant antibiotic exposure in recent years, gut microbiome restoration is a meaningful priority. The interventions with the clearest evidence are dietary: increasing dietary fibre (target 30 to 35 grams per day) from diverse whole-food plant sources, including fermented foods (yoghurt, kefir, kimchi, sauerkraut, and kombucha all have evidence for microbiome diversity improvement), reducing ultra-processed food intake, and achieving the 30 plant species per week target.

Probiotic supplementation has a modest evidence base for specific clinical indications — antibiotic-associated diarrhoea, certain IBS subtypes, and post-antibiotic microbiome recovery — but limited evidence for general wellness. Specific strains matter: Lactobacillus rhamnosus GG and Saccharomyces boulardii have the strongest evidence for antibiotic-associated indications; multi-strain products containing Bifidobacterium and Lactobacillus species have some support for IBS. Generic probiotic supplements without strain specification and third-party quality verification are of limited value.

Layer Three: Advanced Clinical Tools and Emerging Therapies

The third layer of a healthspan stack includes the clinical tools and emerging therapies from Part Three of this book: advanced testing (epigenetic clocks, DUTCH hormonal panels, comprehensive microbiome sequencing), and the evidence-evaluated emerging therapies (NAD+ precursors, senolytics, rapamycin, and specialised peptide protocols). These belong in some stacks — for people with the foundations firmly in place, a clear clinical rationale for advanced assessment or intervention, and access to a clinician with genuine expertise in this space.

They do not belong in everyone's stack, and they certainly do not belong as a first step. The research covered in Chapter Thirteen is honest about where the evidence is strong (GLP-1 agonists for metabolic disease and cardiovascular risk), where it is promising but unproven in humans (senolytics, rapamycin), and where it is largely preclinical with variable human results (most peptide therapies other than GLP-1s).

These are not reasons to dismiss the third layer — they are reasons to approach it with appropriate calibration and clinical oversight.

The guiding question for Layer Three is: given what I know about my starting point, my foundations, and my targeted additions, is there a specific clinical question that can only be answered by an advanced tool or therapy? If the answer is yes, and you have a clinician who can properly order, interpret, and act on the results — then it belongs in your stack. If the answer is no, or if the foundations and targeted additions are still being established, the Layer Three investment is premature.

Building Sustainably: The Time Architecture of Change

One of the most consistent findings in behavioural research is that people systematically overestimate what they can change in a week and underestimate what they can change in a year. The impulse to change everything at once — new exercise programme, new diet, new supplements, new sleep schedule, all starting Monday — is deeply human and almost always counterproductive. The cognitive and practical load of simultaneous large-scale change exceeds most people's bandwidth, leading to rapid deterioration and the painful sense of having failed again.

A more effective approach sequences change over time, building each new behaviour until it becomes genuinely habitual before adding the next. The research on habit formation suggests that new behaviours take between two months and eight months to become automatic, depending on their complexity and how consistently they are practised. Stacking a new behaviour onto an established one — habit stacking — is one of the most reliable methods for building sustainability.

A Practical Sequencing Framework

The following is a suggested time architecture for building a comprehensive healthspan stack. It is a framework, not a prescription. Your starting point, existing habits, life circumstances, and priority gaps will determine the right sequence for you.

Months one and two: Choose one physical activity commitment and one nutritional change, and do nothing else new. The physical activity commitment should be specific, scheduled, and realistic — not 'exercise more' but 'walk for 30 minutes on Monday, Wednesday, and Friday after work.' The nutritional change should address your single largest dietary gap, whether that is protein adequacy, reducing ultra-processed food, or increasing plant diversity. These two changes, done consistently for eight weeks, build the behavioural scaffolding on which everything else rests.

Months three and four: Add resistance training if not already in place (two sessions per week), and begin addressing your sleep priority if this is a significant gap. By this point the aerobic activity is established; adding structured strength work is a manageable expansion. If sleep apnoea investigation is indicated, initiate it now. If insomnia management is needed, begin a CBT-I programme.

Months five and six: Consolidate and optimise. By this point most people have a meaningful aerobic base, a resistance training practice, improved dietary patterns, and better sleep. This is the right time to refine rather than expand: adjust exercise intensity or volume, tighten nutritional specifics, address stress management practices more deliberately. This is also a reasonable time to arrange the core blood panel and functional tests from Chapter Fourteen if you have not already done so — you will have a genuine baseline of improved behaviour to compare future results against.

Months seven to twelve: Based on your test results and the gap analysis from Chapter Fourteen, introduce the targeted additions most relevant to your specific situation. This might mean hormone therapy discussions, a metabolic focus on specific dietary changes, cardiovascular risk management, or specific supplementation. By now the foundations are genuinely solid, and these additions have a stable platform to work from.

Beyond twelve months: Review, adjust, and — for those with the foundations firmly in place and a specific clinical rationale — consider whether any Layer Three tools belong in the plan. By this point you have also lived with your stack long enough to know what is actually working for you, what fits your life, and what needs adapting. No plan survives first contact with reality unchanged, and that is not a failure — it is information.

Supplementation: The Honest Guide

Supplements occupy a peculiar place in the healthspan conversation — simultaneously overhyped by the wellness industry and reflexively dismissed by conventional medicine. The honest position sits between these extremes. Some supplements have a meaningful evidence base for specific indications at specific doses. Many do not. The quality of the evidence for supplements rarely matches what is available for pharmaceutical drugs or lifestyle interventions, partly because there is limited financial incentive to fund the large randomised trials that would settle the questions definitively.

The following is a tiered guide to supplementation based on current evidence strength.

Strong Evidence, Broadly Applicable

- **Vitamin D3 (1,000–2,000 IU daily):** Deficiency is common and has meaningful consequences for bone, immune, and metabolic health. Test first; supplement to achieve serum levels above 75 nmol/L.

- **Omega-3 fatty acids (EPA+DHA, 1–3 grams daily):** Strong evidence for cardiovascular risk reduction at higher doses in people with elevated triglycerides; broad anti-inflammatory benefits at lower doses. Choose quality-verified products (IFOS-certified or equivalent). Algal oil is the plant-based equivalent.

- **Magnesium glycinate or** threonate (300–400 mg elemental, evening): Deficiency is common on Western diets. Supports sleep quality, muscle function, glucose metabolism, and cardiovascular health. Well-tolerated and inexpensive.

- **Creatine monohydrate (3–5 grams daily):** Strong evidence for muscle strength and power gains, particularly in older adults. Emerging evidence for cognitive benefits. Safe across decades of use. One of the most cost-effective supplements in this space.

Good Evidence, More Targeted

- **Collagen peptides (10–15 grams daily, with vitamin C, before exercise):** Growing evidence for joint health, tendon integrity, and skin collagen synthesis in the context of exercise. Most useful for people with joint symptoms or high training loads.

- **Berberine (**500 mg two to three times daily with meals): Reasonable evidence for improving insulin sensitivity, fasting glucose, and lipid markers in people with metabolic dysfunction. Mechanisms overlap with metformin. Not a substitute for medical management of established diabetes.

- **Coenzyme Q10 (100–**200 mg daily, ubiquinol form): Strong evidence for reducing statin-associated myalgia. Reasonable evidence for mild cardiac support in people with heart failure. Less clear benefit for healthy adults without these indications.

- **Probiotics (strain-specific):** Evidence is indication-specific — strongest for antibiotic-associated diarrhoea and certain IBS subtypes. Choose products with documented strain identity and third-party quality verification.

Emerging Evidence, Individual Consideration

- **NMN or NR (250–**500 mg daily): Reliably raises blood NAD+ levels. Modest functional benefits in some trials. Most appropriate for people aged 50+ with confirmed low NAD+ on testing. Use liposomal NMN for superior bioavailability if this is your choice.

- **Fisetin (500–**1,000 mg, intermittent pulsed dosing): Reasonable preclinical senolytic evidence; human safety data is favourable. A low-risk addition for those interested in senolytic approaches without the complexity of dasatinib.

- **Lion's Mane mushroom extract (500–**1,000 mg daily): Promising human trial evidence for nerve growth factor stimulation and mild cognitive improvements, particularly in older adults. Low risk, reasonable rationale for those with cognitive health focus.

- **Ashwagandha (300–**600 mg KSM-66 extract daily): Good RCT evidence for cortisol reduction, stress resilience, and modest improvements in strength and recovery. Useful for people with high chronic stress loads.

Supplements Not Worth the Investment for Most People

Multivitamins, unless correcting confirmed specific deficiencies. Antioxidant megadoses (high-dose vitamin C, vitamin E, beta-carotene), which can paradoxically blunt exercise adaptations. Testosterone boosters and growth hormone precursors marketed to consumers without clinical assessment. Generic collagen drinks without meaningful dose or quality control. And the long list of single-ingredient extracts marketed on the basis of one small pilot study or compelling mechanism arguments with no human trial support.

Your Personal Stack: A Summary Framework

Layer	What It Includes	Who It's For
Layer 1: Foundations	Cardiorespiratory training (150+ min/wk); resistance training (2x/wk); whole-food diet with adequate protein; 7–9 hours quality sleep; stress management; meaningful social connection; not smoking	Everyone. Non-negotiable. Build before adding anything else.
Layer 2: Targeted Additions	Based on priority gaps: metabolic interventions, hormonal therapy, cardiovascular risk management, sleep apnoea treatment, targeted supplementation, cognitive health focus, gut restoration	People with identified gaps from Chapter 14 assessment, with foundations in place.
Layer 3: Advanced Clinical	Advanced testing (epigenetic clocks, DUTCH, Microba); clinical therapies (GLP-1s, MHT, TRT, metformin); emerging therapies (senolytics, rapamycin, NAD+ precursors) under medical supervision	People with solid foundations, specific clinical rationale, and access to experienced clinician.

Tracking Progress: What to Measure and When

A stack without measurement is a program without feedback. You need some way of knowing whether the changes you are making are actually producing biological improvement, or whether you are doing the work without the benefit — which can happen when a key variable (undiagnosed sleep apnoea, untreated hormonal deficiency, sustained high stress) is limiting your adaptive response.

The most important things to track are the measures from your starting point assessment that were most abnormal. If your HOMA-IR was elevated, retest it at six months. If your VO2 max estimate was in the lowest quintile, retest it at six months. If your grip strength was below threshold, track it monthly. If your hs-CRP was above 3.0, retest it at three to six months after dietary and exercise changes.

Track direction, not absolute numbers. A HOMA-IR moving from 4.2 to 2.8 over six months is meaningful progress even if it has not yet reached the optimal range. A VO2 max moving from the lowest to the second-lowest quintile is a clinically significant mortality risk reduction regardless of the absolute value. The direction of travel over time is more informative than the snapshot value at any single measurement.

Do not over-test. Repeating comprehensive bloods every four to six weeks generates data without the signal-to-noise ratio to be clinically useful and creates anxiety without actionable information. A reasonable review rhythm for most people who are making active changes is: functional physical tests every two to three months (these are free and can be done at home); core blood panel every six months for the first year of active change, then annually once stable; and review of your healthspan stack with your GP once a year, or sooner if new symptoms or significant findings emerge.

"Your healthspan stack is not a destination you arrive at. It is a living framework you refine over years — adding what works, removing what does not, adjusting to life's seasons, and holding the foundations steady through all of it."

Chapter Summary

- A healthspan stack is the personalised combination of interventions that work together across your biological systems. It is built in layers, with foundations before targeted additions, and advanced clinical tools only where there is a specific rationale.

- Layer One (foundations) is non-negotiable for everyone: cardiorespiratory and resistance training, whole-food diet with adequate protein and plant diversity, 7–9 hours quality sleep, stress management and social connection, and not smoking. These account for the majority of modifiable healthspan gains available.

- Exercise requires three components to be complete: cardiorespiratory training (VO2 max and cardiovascular protection), resistance training (muscle, bone, and metabolic health), and a combination of zone 2 and HIIT for mitochondrial and metabolic flexibility. Each serves a distinct biological purpose.

- Protein adequacy (1.6–2.2 g/kg/day) is one of the most commonly unmet nutritional needs in the 40–65 age range, with significant consequences for muscle preservation and metabolic health. Plant diversity (30+ species per week) is the single strongest dietary predictor of gut microbiome health.

- Layer Two (targeted additions) is personalised by starting point: metabolic interventions for insulin resistance, hormone therapy for perimenopause and hypogonadism, cardiovascular risk management tools, sleep treatment, and targeted supplementation. These are most effective when the foundations are genuinely in place.

- Layer Three (advanced clinical) includes advanced testing and emerging therapies from Part Three. These belong in stacks with a specific clinical rationale and experienced clinician oversight — not as a first step, and not as a substitute for foundations.

- Supplementation tiers: strong broad evidence (vitamin D, omega-3, magnesium, creatine); good targeted evidence (berberine, CoQ10, collagen, strain-specific probiotics); emerging (NMN/NR, fisetin, lion's mane, ashwagandha). Multivitamins and antioxidant megadoses offer limited value for most people.

- Sustainable change is sequenced, not simultaneous. Two months per new behaviour before adding the next; foundations before targeted additions; review and adjust at six and twelve months based on objective measures.

- Track direction, not absolute numbers, at appropriate intervals: functional physical tests every two to three months; core blood panel every six months during active change, then annually. Over-testing generates anxiety without actionable signal.

Chapter Sixteen

Talking to Your Doctor

I want to begin this chapter with something that might seem obvious but often is not: your doctor works for you. Not in the transactional sense — not the way a plumber works for you, arriving with a fixed toolkit to fix a specific problem and leaving. More in the sense that the entire purpose of the clinical relationship is your health and your life, and that means both of you need to be actively engaged in directing it.

The reality of general practice in Australia in 2025 is that the average GP consultation lasts eleven to thirteen minutes. That is not a criticism of GPs — it is a structural reality of the system they work in, which is chronically underfunded for the complexity of what it is being asked to do. A good GP in that time can diagnose, prescribe, counsel, and refer with extraordinary efficiency and care. But they cannot proactively scan the horizon of your long-term healthspan while simultaneously managing your acute presentation, reviewing your medication list, updating your health summary, and coordinating with three specialists. Much of what this book has covered falls into a category that requires you to bring it into the consultation, not wait for it to be offered.

This chapter is about how to do that effectively. How to have the conversations about healthspan, prevention, and longevity medicine that the standard healthcare system does not always initiate. How to understand what your GP can and cannot help with in a standard consultation, and when specialist referral is warranted. How to navigate the increasingly important world of integrative and longevity medicine in Australia. And how to be an informed, active participant in your own healthcare without falling into the trap of substituting Dr Google for a real clinical relationship.

"The best clinical relationship I have ever seen is one where the patient arrives prepared, the doctor listens properly, and both leave the room knowing exactly what was decided and why. That does not happen by accident. It is the result of both parties taking the conversation seriously."

Understanding What Your GP Can and Cannot Do

Your GP is, in most cases, the most important doctor in your life. They hold longitudinal knowledge of your history, your medications, your family, and your context that no specialist can replicate. They are the coordinator of your care, the person most likely to notice when something does not fit, and the gatekeeper to the investigations and specialist referrals that the system requires. For people who have a long-standing relationship with a GP they trust, this is an enormous asset.

But general practice is structured around episodic, problem-focused consultations. The training, the time, and the Medicare billing structure all align to support acute and chronic disease management, not proactive healthspan optimisation. Many of the topics this book covers — optimising VO2 max, assessing biological ageing, discussing the evidence for MHT in a woman who is not yet symptomatic, ordering fasting insulin alongside a standard lipid panel, exploring peptide therapies — are not part of the standard consultation template. Your GP may be excellent and still not prioritise these topics unless you raise them.

There is also significant variation in how current different GPs are on the topics covered in this book. The evidence base for menopausal hormone therapy has changed substantially since the early 2000s, but some GPs still hold the risk perceptions shaped by the original WHI trial. The evidence for biological age testing is moving faster than many continuing medical education programmes can track. The conversations about insulin resistance, HOMA-IR, and ApoB are becoming more mainstream in proactive medicine but are not yet standard in every practice.

None of this means your GP is the wrong person to talk to — quite the opposite. It means you need to bring these conversations to them informed, specific, and collaborative rather than expecting them to arise spontaneously. It also means that occasionally, for specific topics, you may need access to a clinician with more specialised expertise in the particular area you are pursuing.

Preparing for the Conversation

The most productive healthspan conversations I have seen happen when the patient has done three things before walking in the door: decided what they want from this specific appointment, prepared the relevant information, and thought about what questions they genuinely want answered. This sounds simple, but most people arrive at a GP consultation with a vague sense of what they want to discuss and leave without having covered the most important things because the consultation drifted in other directions.

Decide What You Want From This Appointment

Be specific. 'I want to talk about my health' is not a goal for an eleven-minute consultation. 'I want to discuss ordering a fasting insulin and ApoB alongside my usual annual bloods, and I want to understand my cardiovascular risk based on what those results show' is a goal. 'I have been reading about the updated evidence on menopausal hormone therapy and I want to understand whether it is appropriate for me given my personal history' is a goal. One or two specific goals per appointment is realistic. Five is not.

If your GP offers extended consultations (typically 30 to 40 minutes, billed under a different Medicare item number), booking one of these for a comprehensive healthspan review is worth doing once a year. Mention when you book that you want a health review, not just a prescription renewal — this gives the GP time to prepare and ensures the consultation is structured appropriately.

Bring the Relevant Information

Bring any recent blood results you have. Bring a list of your current medications and supplements (many people are surprised what they have accumulated). Bring any wearable data that is clinically relevant — resting heart rate trends, sleep duration data, VO2 max estimates from a device. If you have done any testing outside the standard Medicare-rebatable panel — a DUTCH test, a microbiome assessment, an epigenetic age test — bring the reports and be clear that you are seeking clinical interpretation, not just validation.

A brief written summary of your current situation — two or three sentences about what you are trying to address and what you already know — handed to the GP at the start of the consultation is one of the most effective tools I know for ensuring a productive appointment. It gives the GP the context they need immediately and signals that you are prepared and specific, which most clinicians genuinely appreciate.

Know What Questions You Want Answered

Write them down beforehand and have the list with you. The questions that are genuinely most useful are specific and clinical: 'My fasting insulin came back at 18 mIU/L, which I understand is elevated. What does that mean for my cardiovascular risk and what should I do about it?' Not: 'Is insulin resistance bad?' 'I have been experiencing significant sleep disruption for the past six months. I wonder whether this could be related to perimenopause and I would like to understand my options, including the current evidence on hormone therapy.' Not: 'Am I going through menopause?'

If there is something on your question list that you do not get to in the consultation, ask for a follow-up appointment or ask whether your GP is comfortable receiving a brief written query through the practice's patient portal. Many practices now offer this and it is an underused resource for non-urgent clinical questions.

Specific Conversations Worth Having

The following are the conversations that the patients I see most benefit from having with their GP — and that are most often not happening unless the patient initiates them.

The Metabolic Health Conversation

If you have not had a comprehensive metabolic assessment including fasting insulin and HOMA-IR, this is the conversation to initiate. The request is straightforward: 'I understand that standard lipid and glucose panels can miss early insulin resistance. I would like to add fasting insulin to my next blood test so we can calculate HOMA-IR, and I would also like to include ApoB as a more accurate measure of atherogenic particle burden. Can we do that?'

In most Australian general practices, fasting insulin is rebatable on Medicare with appropriate clinical indication (which includes family history of type 2 diabetes, overweight, or symptoms of metabolic syndrome). ApoB may require a private request depending on the laboratory and indication. Discussing this with your GP will establish what is covered in your specific situation.

If your results show elevated HOMA-IR (above 2.5 is suggestive, above 3.5 is clearly abnormal), elevated TG/HDL ratio (above 3.5 is concerning), or waist circumference above clinical thresholds, ask explicitly: 'What is my current trajectory? What are the specific interventions most likely to improve these markers? And at what point would you consider pharmacological options like metformin?' These are reasonable, evidence-grounded questions that your GP should be able to engage with.

The Cardiovascular Risk Conversation

Ask your GP to calculate your absolute cardiovascular risk using the Australian cardiovascular risk calculator (based on the Framingham equation or the newer AusDRisk derivatives), which combines age, sex, smoking status, blood pressure, lipid levels, and family history into a ten-year risk estimate. Understanding your risk number — not just whether individual markers are in range — gives both of you a shared framework for decisions about intervention intensity.

If you have a family history of premature cardiovascular disease (heart attack or stroke in a first-degree male relative before 55, or female relative before 65), ask about coronary artery calcium (CAC) scoring. This is a low-radiation CT scan of the heart that provides a direct measure of subclinical atherosclerosis — the actual accumulation of calcium in arterial plaques — that can identify high-risk individuals years before events occur. It is not available through Medicare for primary prevention screening, but can be accessed privately for approximately $150 to $250 and is among the most informative single tests available for cardiovascular risk stratification. Ask your GP whether it is appropriate in your specific situation.

The Hormonal Health Conversation for Women

If you are in or approaching perimenopause and experiencing symptoms — sleep disruption, hot flushes, mood changes, cognitive fogginess, genitourinary symptoms, or changes in your menstrual cycle — this is the conversation to have: 'I have been reading about the updated evidence on menopausal hormone therapy, particularly about the difference in risk profile between older oral synthetic hormones and the newer transdermal and body-identical formulations. Can we discuss whether MHT is appropriate for me, and if so, what formulation you would recommend?'

Some GPs are highly current on the evidence and will engage immediately with a nuanced discussion about transdermal oestradiol and micronised progesterone. Others may hold more cautious views shaped by the original WHI trial and may need more time to engage with the updated data. If you feel your concerns are being dismissed rather than engaged with, a referral to a gynaecologist or a specialist in menopause medicine is entirely appropriate. Menopause societies in Australia publish guidelines and maintain lists of practitioners with specific menopause expertise.

For women with significant symptoms, the question of MHT should not be closed without a genuine clinical discussion. The evidence is clear that for most healthy women under 60 who are within ten years of menopause, the benefits of properly prescribed MHT substantially outweigh the risks. You deserve a clinician who is current on that evidence.

The Hormonal Health Conversation for Men

If you are experiencing symptoms consistent with low testosterone — persistent fatigue, reduced libido, difficulty maintaining muscle mass despite exercise, mood changes, reduced morning erections, or cognitive changes — ask for a testosterone assessment: 'I have been experiencing several symptoms that may be related to declining testosterone. Can we do a morning fasting total testosterone, free testosterone, and SHBG to get a complete picture?'

Two morning fasting measurements are required to confirm a low result, as testosterone varies across the day and day to day. If results are consistently below normal reference ranges and symptoms are present, a discussion about the options — including whether TRT is appropriate, what monitoring would be required, and what the risks and benefits are in your specific situation — is warranted. Your GP may refer you to an endocrinologist or a urologist with specific andrology expertise for this conversation.

The Sleep Conversation

If you snore regularly, your partner has observed breathing pauses during sleep, or you consistently wake unrefreshed despite adequate sleep opportunity, ask specifically: 'I think I may have sleep apnoea. Can we arrange a home sleep study?' Home sleep studies can be arranged through most GP practices and are Medicare-rebatable for patients with clinical features of obstructive sleep apnoea. The result directly informs treatment, which — if significant apnoea is confirmed — is among the highest-impact interventions available.

If insomnia is the issue — difficulty falling or staying asleep, not sleep apnoea — ask specifically about Cognitive Behavioural Therapy for Insomnia (CBT-I) referral or validated digital CBT-I programmes, rather than accepting a sleeping medication prescription as the first-line response. CBT-I is more effective than medication for chronic insomnia long-term. Your GP may refer you to a psychologist with sleep specialisation, or be aware of specific CBT-I digital programmes with good evidence behind them.

The Bone Health Conversation

For women over 50 and men over 60 — and for anyone with a history of significant weight loss, high corticosteroid use, or early menopause — a DEXA scan for bone mineral density provides important baseline information about fracture risk. Ask: 'Given my age and history, is a DEXA scan for bone mineral density appropriate? I would like to understand where I stand and whether there are specific interventions I should be making.' DEXA scans are Medicare-rebatable in specific circumstances; your GP can advise on eligibility. Bone health is a silent issue until it is not — the fracture that changes everything is a preventable event for many people with the right information and appropriate early intervention.

The Mental Health Conversation

Depression, anxiety, and burnout are not inevitable features of midlife, and they are not weakness. They are treatable medical conditions with meaningful consequences for physical health, biological ageing, cognitive function, and quality of life. The mortality risk associated with untreated depression is significant and frequently underappreciated in the context of physical health discussions.

If you have persistent low mood, significant anxiety, loss of enjoyment in activities that previously engaged you, or feel chronically overwhelmed in ways that are not improving with rest, raise it directly: 'I have been experiencing persistent low mood and I would like to discuss whether this warrants assessment and treatment.' Effective treatments exist — psychological therapies, medication where indicated, and in some cases assessment for underlying contributors like thyroid dysfunction, low testosterone, or vitamin D deficiency — and the right clinician will take this seriously.

Navigating the Broader Healthcare System

When to Ask for a Specialist Referral

Your GP is the appropriate first port of call for all of the conversations above, and most can be handled within the GP-patient relationship. But there are situations where specialist expertise adds meaningful value that a generalist cannot replicate.

Consider asking for a referral to a cardiologist or preventive cardiologist if: your absolute cardiovascular risk is high (above 15 to 20 per cent over ten years); your CAC score is significantly elevated; you have concerning findings on resting ECG; or you have a strong family history of premature cardiovascular disease and want a comprehensive risk assessment from a specialist.

Consider a referral to an endocrinologist if: testosterone results are consistently low and your GP is not comfortable managing TRT; thyroid findings are complex or symptoms are not resolving with standard management; adrenal or pituitary abnormalities are suspected; or metabolic disease management requires specialist input.

Consider a referral to a gynaecologist with menopause expertise if: your GP is not current on MHT evidence or is unwilling to discuss it; you have a complex history (prior breast cancer, clotting disorders, or other contraindications) that requires specialist risk assessment; or you want to discuss surgical menopause management or more complex hormonal scenarios.

Consider a referral to a sleep physician or respiratory physician if: home sleep study results suggest significant obstructive sleep apnoea (AHI above 15 events per hour); CPAP compliance is poor and alternatives need assessment; or complex sleep disorders beyond straightforward OSA are suspected.

Consider a referral to an exercise physiologist if: you have musculoskeletal limitations, cardiovascular conditions, metabolic disease, or any situation where supervised exercise prescription would reduce injury risk and improve outcomes. Exercise physiologists in Australia are university-trained allied health professionals with specific expertise in exercise as medicine; they are not gym trainers.

Integrative and Longevity Medicine in Australia

A growing number of medical practitioners in Australia describe themselves as practicing integrative medicine, functional medicine, or longevity medicine. These terms are not precisely regulated, and the quality and evidence-orientation of practitioners in this space varies significantly. At its best, integrative and longevity medicine represents exactly the kind of proactive, whole-person, prevention-focused care that this book has been describing. At its worst, it represents expensive consultations with extensive testing that generates data without clear clinical implications, and recommendations that are not grounded in the evidence hierarchy described in Chapter Thirteen.

The questions worth asking before engaging with any practitioner in this space are the same questions you would apply to any clinical recommendation: What is the evidence for this? Is the evidence from human clinical trials, animal studies, or mechanism arguments? What are the known risks and unknowns? Is the cost proportionate to the expected benefit? Is this practitioner registered with AHPRA and operating within their scope of practice?

A good integrative or longevity medicine practitioner will welcome these questions. They will be honest about where the evidence is strong and where it is emerging. They will not recommend investigations or treatments that cannot be justified by the evidence to an informed patient. They will have a clear framework for prioritisation — foundations before complexity — rather than immediately reaching for the most elaborate and expensive intervention.

Red flags in this space include: practitioners who recommend extensive testing panels without clear clinical questions being asked; those who recommend large numbers of supplements without individual clinical justification; those who are dismissive of conventional medicine or who frame everything in terms of 'what your regular doctor won't tell you'; and those whose revenue model depends heavily on selling products alongside clinical advice. These patterns do not automatically indicate a bad practitioner, but they warrant careful evaluation.

The Role of Allied Health

Some of the most high-impact interventions available in healthspan medicine are delivered not by doctors but by allied health professionals — and they are significantly underused in the 40 to 65 age range.

Exercise physiologists, as noted above, can design safe and effective exercise programmes for people with specific health conditions or rehabilitation needs that a generic gym programme cannot address.

Dietitians with experience in metabolic health or sports nutrition can translate the nutritional principles in this book into a practical, personalised eating plan that accounts for your preferences, schedule, and specific health goals.

Psychologists and psychological therapists provide CBT-I for insomnia, acceptance and commitment therapy or cognitive behavioural therapy for chronic stress and anxiety, and support for the behavioural change process that underlies sustainable lifestyle modification. The mindset and behavioural skills covered in Chapter Eight are genuinely learnable with support, and a good psychologist is one of the highest-leverage investments available in this space.

Physiotherapists can address the musculoskeletal limitations — chronic pain, restricted mobility, joint problems — that frequently prevent people from building the exercise foundation that everything else depends on. Many people in their forties and fifties have accumulated musculoskeletal issues that are genuinely addressable with appropriate assessment and treatment, but which have been normalised as 'just ageing.'

All of the above allied health services are accessible with or without GP referral, and many are partially rebatable through Medicare chronic disease management plans (CDM plans, formerly Enhanced Primary Care plans) where your GP can arrange up to five rebated allied health sessions per year for patients with chronic health conditions.

Being an Informed Patient Without Being a Difficult One

There is a version of the informed, proactive patient who drives their doctor to distraction: the one who arrives with a printed stack of studies, challenges every recommendation, and has already decided what treatment they want before the consultation begins. That is not what this chapter is advocating.

Being informed means understanding enough to ask good questions, not enough to bypass clinical judgement. It means arriving with relevant information, not arriving with a diagnosis. It means being able to say 'I have read that fasting insulin is a more sensitive marker of insulin resistance than fasting glucose — is there a clinical reason not to include it in my panel?' rather than 'I want fasting insulin ordered.' The difference is subtle but important: the first invites clinical engagement; the second creates a dynamic where the clinician is being directed rather than consulted.

Most clinicians respond well to patients who have done their homework, are specific about what they want, and are genuinely interested in understanding the clinical reasoning rather than just receiving a recommendation. The patients I have most enjoyed working with across a career spanning pharmacy and medicine are exactly this kind of person: curious, prepared, and collaborative. They make me better at my job because they hold me to a higher standard of explanation and engagement.

The one area where directness is unambiguously appropriate is when you feel your concerns are not being taken seriously. If you raise a symptom or concern and it is dismissed without adequate explanation, it is entirely reasonable to say: 'I understand you may not be concerned, but this is something I feel is affecting my quality of life and I would like to explore it further. Can we discuss what investigation would be appropriate, or whether a referral makes sense?' Persistence in the face of genuine symptoms is not being difficult. It is advocating for your own health.

Practical Guide: Conversations and Who to Have Them With

Topic	What to Ask	Who	Notes
Metabolic panel	Add fasting insulin, HOMA-IR, ApoB to annual bloods	GP	Fasting insulin rebatable with clinical indication

Topic	What to Ask	Who	Notes
Cardiovascular risk	Calculate absolute 10-year CV risk; discuss CAC scan if appropriate	GP → Cardiologist if high risk	CAC scan private ~$150–250
Perimenopause / MHT	Discuss updated MHT evidence; explore transdermal oestradiol + micronised progesterone	GP or Gynaecologist	Refer if GP not current on evidence
Low testosterone	Morning fasting testosterone x2, free T, SHBG; discuss TRT if confirmed low	GP → Endocrinologist or Urologist	Requires two measurements to confirm
Sleep apnoea	Arrange home sleep study; discuss CPAP if AHI >15	GP → Sleep Physician	Medicare-rebatable home study with clinical indication
Insomnia	Request CBT-I referral rather than sleep medication as first line	GP → Psychologist	5 CDM-rebated sessions/yr available
Bone density	DEXA scan if age + risk factors present	GP → Radiologist	Medicare-rebatable in specific circumstances

Topic	What to Ask	Who	Notes
Mental health	Raise persistent mood, anxiety or burnout directly; explore treatment options	GP → Psychologist or Psychiatrist	CDM plan available; Mental Health Care Plan
Exercise prescription	Safe exercise programme with health conditions or rehab needs	Exercise Physiologist	CDM rebate available
Nutritional planning	Personalised eating plan for metabolic or body composition goals	Dietitian	CDM rebate available
Musculoskel etal issues	Assessment and treatment of pain or mobility limitations blocking exercise	Physiotherapi st	Private or CDM rebate

A Final Word on the Clinical Relationship

Medicine works best when it is a genuine partnership. Your clinicians bring training, clinical pattern recognition, and access to investigations and treatments that you cannot provide for yourself. You bring knowledge of your own experience, your history, your values, and your willingness to engage with the changes that improve health. Neither half of that partnership is complete without the other.

The healthcare system in Australia, for all its imperfections, is one of the best in the world at managing acute and chronic disease. Where it is weaker — and where this book has tried to fill some of the gap — is in the proactive, longitudinal, whole-person approach to healthspan that the evidence increasingly supports. That gap is closing, slowly, as the culture of medicine shifts and as more practitioners develop expertise in preventive and longevity medicine. But in the meantime, you do not have to wait for the system to catch up.

You can arrive informed. You can ask good questions. You can advocate for investigations and conversations that the evidence supports. You can build a team of clinicians and allied health professionals who collectively cover the domains that matter for your long-term health. And you can approach the whole enterprise with the understanding that your health is not something that happens to you — it is something you participate in creating, every day, through the choices this book has tried to illuminate.

"The most important appointment in preventive medicine is not the one where a disease is caught early. It is the conversation that happens years before, where a person and their doctor look at the trajectory together and decide, deliberately, to redirect it."

Chapter Summary

- The average Australian GP consultation is eleven to thirteen minutes — sufficient for skilled acute and chronic disease management, but not for proactive healthspan conversations unless you initiate them. Arrive prepared, specific, and with clear goals.

- Preparing for a productive consultation means: deciding one or two specific goals for the appointment, bringing relevant test results and medication/supplement lists, and writing down your key questions beforehand.

- The metabolic health conversation (fasting insulin, HOMA-IR, ApoB) is the most commonly missed clinical assessment for people aged 40 to 65. It requires initiating, not waiting. Fasting insulin is Medicare-rebatable with appropriate clinical indication.

- The cardiovascular risk conversation should include absolute risk calculation (ten-year risk) and, for people with significant family history or multiple risk factors, a discussion about coronary artery calcium scoring as a direct measure of subclinical atherosclerosis.

- The MHT conversation for perimenopausal women deserves a GP who is current on the post-WHI evidence. If yours is not, a referral to a gynaecologist with menopause expertise is appropriate. The evidence strongly supports MHT for most symptomatic women under 60 within ten years of menopause.

- Sleep apnoea is dramatically underdiagnosed. If you snore, wake unrefreshed, or have breathing pauses observed, ask for a home sleep study. Treatment of significant sleep apnoea is one of the most impactful preventive interventions available.

- Insomnia should be addressed first with CBT-I referral to a psychologist, not with sleeping medication as the default. CBT-I is more effective long-term. Five rebated sessions per year are available under the Medicare chronic disease management pathway.

- Allied health professionals — exercise physiologists, dietitians, psychologists, and physiotherapists — deliver some of the highest-impact healthspan interventions and are significantly underused. Chronic disease management plans provide up to five rebated sessions per year with GP referral.

- Integrative and longevity medicine practitioners vary enormously in evidence-orientation and quality. Apply the same scrutiny to their recommendations as to any clinical advice: what is the evidence, from what level of the hierarchy, and is the cost proportionate to the expected benefit?

- Being an informed, proactive patient means arriving prepared and asking good questions — not arriving with a predetermined diagnosis or treatment plan. The goal is clinical engagement, not clinical direction. Most clinicians welcome well-prepared, genuinely curious patients.

- If your concerns are dismissed without adequate explanation, it is appropriate to persist. Advocating clearly for investigation of genuine symptoms is not being difficult. It is participating in your own healthcare.

The Long Game

What it means to play for the decades ahead

There is a photograph that I keep in my mind when I think about why I wrote this book. It is not an image of a laboratory, or a clinical trial, or a chart showing the mortality benefit of VO2 max improvement. It is an image of my patients — the ones who have genuinely changed the trajectory of their biological ageing — ten or fifteen years after we started working together. What strikes me most is not what they can no longer do. It is what they still can. They are still hiking. Still playing with grandchildren on the floor and getting back up without a second thought. Still working in ways that feel purposeful rather than grinding. Still curious, still engaged, still themselves.

That is what healthspan actually means in practice. Not a number on an epigenetic clock, although those matter. Not a VO2 max percentile, although that matters too. It is the preservation of the things that make a life feel worth living — physical capacity, cognitive clarity, emotional resilience, meaningful connection — into the decades when those things are most easily surrendered.

The science that underpins this book is genuinely exciting. We are living through an era of extraordinary progress in our understanding of how ageing works at the biological level, and that understanding is beginning to translate into practical tools for intervention. But the most important message of this book is not about any of those tools. It is far simpler.

The biology of ageing is not a passive process that happens to you. It is a dynamic system that responds — throughout your entire adult life, and with more plasticity than most people realise — to how you live. The choices you make about how you move, what you eat, how you sleep, how you manage stress, how you invest in your relationships, and how you engage with the healthcare system are not peripheral to your biology. They are your biology. They are the upstream inputs that determine the downstream outputs: the inflammatory load, the epigenetic age, the insulin sensitivity, the cognitive reserve, the muscle mass and bone density that will either support or constrain your life in the decades to come.

This is both sobering and enormously liberating. Sobering because it means there is no passive path to a good healthspan. Liberating because it means the trajectory is modifiable — at almost any starting point, and often more rapidly than people expect.

"The most powerful intervention in longevity medicine is not a drug, a supplement, or a test. It is the sustained, daily decision to live in a way that your future self will benefit from."

What the Evidence Actually Tells Us

Across sixteen chapters, this book has covered a great deal of ground. The biological mechanisms of ageing, the foundations of physical health and nutrition, the evidence on sleep, stress, hormones, gut health, and metabolic function, the emerging therapies that may one day extend what is possible, and the practical frameworks for building a personalised healthspan plan and navigating the healthcare system effectively. It is worth pausing to distil what the evidence, taken as a whole, most clearly says.

It says that physical fitness — cardiorespiratory fitness in particular — is the single most powerful modifiable predictor of how long and how well you will live. More powerful than any medication, any supplement, any emerging therapy. Moving from the bottom fitness quintile to the second-lowest quintile reduces all-cause mortality by more than eliminating smoking. This single finding should reshape how we think about exercise: not as a lifestyle choice or a cosmetic pursuit, but as the most essential medical intervention available.

It says that the metabolic diseases driving the most years lost to disability and premature death — type 2 diabetes, cardiovascular disease, and increasingly dementia — are largely preventable and in many cases reversible, given sufficiently early and sufficiently sustained lifestyle intervention. The insulin resistance that underlies most of these conditions begins a decade or more before clinical diagnosis. The window for intervention is not a brief crisis moment. It is a long, quiet opportunity that most people do not recognise as such because nothing yet hurts.

It says that sleep is not negotiable. That the chronic sleep deprivation normalised in modern professional and parenting life extracts a measurable biological cost that no supplement or exercise programme can compensate for. And that addressing poor sleep — whether through behavioural change, sleep apnoea treatment, or in some cases hormonal management — is among the highest-leverage improvements available to most adults in the 40 to 65 age range.

It says that the brain is not a fixed organ that inevitably deteriorates with age. It is a dynamic, responsive tissue that benefits from cardiovascular health, metabolic regulation, sleep, stress management, novel learning, and social engagement, and that the choices made in midlife have measurable consequences for cognitive function and dementia risk decades later.

And it says, with unusual consistency across every domain, that the foundations matter more than the additions. Exercise, nutrition, sleep, stress management, and social connection are not the boring prerequisites while you wait for the interesting interventions. They are the intervention. The emerging therapies of Chapter Thirteen are genuinely promising, and some of them will prove transformative. But none of them operate in a biological vacuum. They work best — some of them only work at all — in a biological environment created by the foundations.

The Patient I Want You to Be

Across a career that has spanned pharmacy and medicine, I have watched thousands of patients make choices about their health — choices that compounded, slowly and invisibly, into the state of their bodies and their lives a decade later. The patients who have done best are not the ones who were born with the most genetic advantage, or who had access to the most sophisticated tests and therapies. They are the ones who decided, usually at some turning point in midlife, to take their future health seriously enough to act on the evidence.

They asked questions. They got the tests their standard annual checks were missing. They brought the relevant information to their doctors and had the conversations the system does not always initiate. They built exercise into their lives not as a heroic effort but as a non-negotiable structure. They changed the way they ate — not dramatically or punitively, but decisively. They addressed the sleep problem they had been tolerating for years. They took their mental health as seriously as their physical health. And they adjusted, year after year, as they learned more about what was actually working.

That is the patient I want this book to help you become. Not a passive recipient of whatever care the system delivers. Not an anxious optimiser chasing the perfect biomarker score. But an informed, engaged, proactive person who understands enough about their own biology to make good decisions, ask the right questions, and build — patiently, persistently, over years — a life that is as healthy as the science and your circumstances allow.

A Final Word on Time

There is one more thing worth saying, and it is perhaps the most important.

The research on healthspan is full of astonishing numbers. The mortality benefit of moving from one fitness quintile to another. The epigenetic age reversal achievable with sustained lifestyle change. The reduction in dementia risk associated with decades of exercise and healthy eating. These numbers are real, and they are motivating. But they can also make the whole enterprise feel monumental — as though the only meaningful action is a complete overhaul, beginning immediately and maintained perfectly forever.

That is not how any of this actually works. Meaningful biological change begins with the first consistent step, not the perfect plan. A person who walks briskly three times a week for six months has a meaningfully different cardiovascular and metabolic biology than the person who planned to run a marathon but has not started yet. A person who eats two additional serves of vegetables a day and reduces their alcohol intake from five nights a week to two has a measurably different inflammatory load than the one still waiting for the right moment to change everything.

The biology does not require heroism. It requires consistency. And consistency does not require perfection — it requires direction. As long as you are moving in the right direction, with more good weeks than bad ones, learning from what does and does not work for you, and building the habits that compound over time, you are doing the work.

You have more time than you think. And the biology you build between now and the end of that time matters more than almost anything else you will spend that time on.

Begin.

> *"The decade between 45 and 55 is not a waiting room. It is one of the most important periods of biological investment available in a human life. What you build there — in fitness, in metabolic health, in cognitive reserve, in social connection — is what you will live from for the decades that follow."*

—

Appendix A: Key Blood Tests and Reference Ranges

The following tables summarise the blood markers most relevant to healthspan assessment, with reference ranges as used in standard Australian clinical practice and the optimal ranges used in proactive medicine. Where these differ, both are listed. All values should be interpreted in the clinical context of the individual, and results outside optimal ranges should be discussed with your GP.

Marker	Standard Reference Range	Optimal Range (Proactive)	Clinical Notes
Fasting glucose	3.9–5.5 mmol/L	4.0–5.0 mmol/L	Values 5.5–6.9 = prediabetes territory; warrants fasting insulin

Marker	Standard Reference Range	Optimal Range (Proactive)	Clinical Notes
HbA1c	<41 mmol/mol (<5.9%)	<38 mmol/mol (<5.6%)	42–47 = prediabetes; ≥48 = diabetes. Misses early insulin resistance
Fasting insulin	3–25 mIU/L (lab range)	<10 mIU/L (optimal)	High fasting insulin precedes glucose abnormality by years. Calculate HOMA-IR
HOMA-IR	<2.5 (approximate)	<1.5 (optimal)	HOMA-IR = (Fasting insulin x Fasting glucose) / 22.5. Above 3.5 = significant IR
Triglycerides	<2.0 mmol/L	<1.1 mmol/L	Fasting value. Elevated TG with low HDL is the metabolic syndrome signature
HDL cholesterol	>1.0 mmol/L (M) >1.2 mmol/L (F)	>1.6 mmol/L	Higher is better. Low HDL + high TG = elevated cardiovascular and metabolic risk

Marker	Standard Reference Range	Optimal Range (Proactive)	Clinical Notes
TG/HDL ratio	<3.5 (approximate)	<1.5 (optimal)	Strong surrogate for insulin resistance and small dense LDL burden
ApoB	<1.0 g/L (standard)	<0.7 g/L (optimal)	Direct measure of atherogenic particle number. Superior CV risk marker to LDL-C
hs-CRP	<5 mg/L (standard)	<1.0 mg/L (optimal)	Values 1–3 = moderate CV risk; >3 = elevated chronic inflammation. Recheck if >10
Vitamin D (25-OH)	>50 nmol/L (sufficient)	75–150 nmol/L	Deficiency is common in Australian office workers despite climate. Supplement if <75
TSH (thyroid)	0.5–4.5 mIU/L	1.0–2.5 mIU/L	TSH at upper end of range may be functionally low in symptomatic patients. Add fT3/fT4

Marker	Standard Reference Range	Optimal Range (Proactive)	Clinical Notes
Total testosterone (M)	8–30 nmol/L	>15 nmol/L (symptomatic consideration)	Morning fasting sample. Repeat if low. Add SHBG and free T for complete picture
Ferritin	30–300 µg/L (M) 20–200 µg/L (F)	50–150 µg/L	Low = iron deficiency; high = inflammation marker or iron overload (check transferrin sat)

Appendix B: Functional Age Tests — How to Do Them

The following physical tests can all be performed at home or in any GP clinic without specialist equipment. They provide meaningful baseline data and respond to training over weeks to months. Test and record your results, then retest every two to three months.

Single-Leg Balance Test

- Stand barefoot on a hard floor near a wall (for safety if needed)
- Lift one foot and rest it against the calf of the standing leg
- Release your hands from any support and start timing

- Record the longest hold on each side (aim for 10 seconds or more)
- Eyes open. Do not allow the free foot to touch the ground or the standing leg
- Normal: 10+ seconds on each side under age 70. Less than 10 seconds warrants attention at any age under 70

Five-Times Sit-to-Stand Test (STS)

- Use a standard chair (approximately 43–45 cm seat height), against a wall
- Sit with arms folded across your chest — do not use your arms to assist
- On 'go', rise to full standing and sit back down five times as quickly as possible
- Record the total time for five complete repetitions
- Under 12 seconds: good functional performance for adults in their 50s
- 12–15 seconds: fair; 15–17 seconds: some functional decline; above 17 seconds: significant concern

Sitting-Rising Test (SRT)

- From a standing position on a firm carpeted floor, lower yourself to sit cross-legged without using hands, knees, forearms, or any support
- Then rise back to standing without support
- Scoring: start at 10 (5 for sitting, 5 for rising). Subtract 1 for each use of a hand, knee, or forearm. Subtract 0.5 for any significant loss of balance
- Score 8–10: excellent. 6–7: good. Below 6: meaningful functional limitation

- This test is harder than it looks and most adults are surprised by their result

Grip Strength (with dynamometer)

- If using a hand dynamometer: stand with arm at side, elbow slightly bent, squeeze as hard as possible for 3–5 seconds
- Record the peak reading. Test both hands, alternate three times, take the best result
- Men: above 40 kg = excellent; 30–40 kg = good; 26–30 kg = acceptable; below 26 kg = clinically low
- Women: above 25 kg = excellent; 20–25 kg = good; 16–20 kg = acceptable; below 16 kg = clinically low
- Thresholds sourced from international sarcopenia diagnostic criteria (EWGSOP2)

Appendix C: A Note on Navigating Further Information

The field of longevity and healthspan medicine moves quickly. What follows is a brief guide to navigating the information landscape, and to distinguishing sources likely to produce accurate, evidence-grounded information from those likely to produce noise.

High-Quality Primary Sources

For those who want to go deeper into the primary scientific literature, the following databases provide free access to abstracts and, increasingly, full-text articles:

- **PubMed (pubmed.ncbi.nlm.nih.gov):** The US National Library of Medicine's database of biomedical literature. The best starting point for any specific clinical question. Use the filters to identify review articles and clinical trials specifically.

- **Cochrane Library (cochranelibrary.com):** Systematic reviews and meta-analyses of clinical interventions. The most reliable source for evidence-based clinical recommendations. Particularly useful for supplement and intervention questions.

- **The Lancet, NEJM, JAMA, BMJ, Nature Medicine:** The highest-tier peer-reviewed medical journals. Many articles are behind paywalls, but abstracts are always free and often contain the key findings.

Credible Secondary Sources

For well-synthesised, accessible explanations of primary research:

- **Examine.com:** Rigorous, unbiased summaries of supplement and nutrition research. No commercial bias. Each substance has a summary of human evidence with confidence ratings. The best single resource for supplement questions.

- **FoundMyFitness (foundmyfitness.com):** Dr Rhonda Patrick's research-focused content on exercise, nutrition, and ageing. Heavily evidence-grounded and well-referenced. More technical than most consumer health content.

- **The Proof Podcast (theproofpodcast.com):** Simon Hill's long-form interviews with researchers in nutrition and longevity. High evidence standards and willingness to engage with nuance and complexity.

- **Peter Attia's work (peterattia.com):** Particularly his writing on cardiovascular risk, metabolic health, and exercise physiology. Well-referenced, clinically focused, and willing to disagree with mainstream guidance where the evidence supports it.

Australian-Specific Resources

- **Healthdirect (healthdirect.gov.au):** Australian Government-funded health information service. Accurate, clinician-reviewed general health information with Australian context for medications, referrals, and services.

- **NPS MedicineWise (nps.org.au):** Independent, evidence-based information on medicines and medical tests. Particularly useful for medication questions and for understanding what Medicare covers.

- **Jean Hailes Foundation (jeanhailes.org.au):** The leading Australian resource for women's health, including a comprehensive and evidence-current menopause section. Regularly updated.

- **Andrology Australia (andrologyaustralia.org):** The leading Australian resource for men's reproductive and hormonal health, including testosterone assessment and replacement guidance.

Red Flags in Health Information

The following patterns should prompt significant scepticism in any health information source, regardless of how authoritative it sounds:

- Claims that a single intervention, supplement, or test can address multiple unrelated health conditions simultaneously

- Framing that positions the source as having information 'your doctor won't tell you'

- Evidence cited only from animal studies, mechanism arguments, or testimonials, without human clinical trial data

- Commercial products being sold by the same source providing the clinical information

- Absolute claims (always, never, guaranteed) in an area where the science shows dose-dependence, individual variation, and ongoing uncertainty

- Sources that do not distinguish between different grades of evidence — treating a single pilot study the same as a large randomised controlled trial

Appendix D: Glossary of Key Terms

The following terms appear throughout this book. They are defined here for easy reference.

Term	Definition
ApoB	Apolipoprotein B. A protein found on atherogenic lipoproteins (LDL, VLDL, IDL). ApoB count is a direct measure of atherogenic particle number and is a superior cardiovascular risk marker to LDL cholesterol.
Biological age	An estimate of how old an individual's body is at the cellular and molecular level, based on biomarkers rather than years since birth. Typically assessed using epigenetic clocks or functional measures.

Term	Definition
CBT-I	Cognitive Behavioural Therapy for Insomnia. The evidence-based first-line treatment for chronic insomnia, more effective long-term than sleep medication.
DunedinPACE	A third-generation epigenetic clock measuring the pace of biological ageing (how fast someone is ageing) rather than their current biological age.
DUTCH test	Dried Urine Test for Comprehensive Hormones. A comprehensive hormone test using dried urine samples that assesses oestrogen metabolites, cortisol patterns, progesterone, androgens, and other markers.
Epigenetic clock	An algorithm that estimates biological age from patterns of DNA methylation across multiple genomic sites. GrimAge and PhenoAge are the most clinically validated examples.
GLP-1 agonist	Glucagon-like peptide-1 receptor agonist. A class of drugs that mimic the hormone GLP-1, reducing appetite, improving glucose control, and producing significant cardiovascular and metabolic benefits. Examples: semaglutide (Ozempic), tirzepatide (Mounjaro).

Term	Definition
Hallmarks of ageing	The twelve interconnected biological processes identified by López-Otín et al. as the primary drivers of ageing, including genomic instability, telomere attrition, epigenetic alterations, mitochondrial dysfunction, and cellular senescence.
Healthspan	The portion of lifespan spent in good health, free from significant chronic disease or disability. The primary goal of longevity medicine is extending healthspan, not just lifespan.
HOMA-IR	Homeostatic Model Assessment of Insulin Resistance. Calculated as (fasting insulin x fasting glucose) / 22.5. A measure of insulin resistance; values above 2.5 suggest developing resistance, above 3.5 is clearly abnormal.
hs-CRP	High-sensitivity C-reactive protein. An inflammatory marker used to assess cardiovascular risk and chronic systemic inflammation. Values below 1 mg/L are optimal; above 3 mg/L indicates elevated chronic inflammation.
Inflammageing	The chronic, low-grade inflammation that develops with ageing and drives accelerated deterioration across multiple organ systems. A major contributor to cardiovascular disease, dementia, cancer, and frailty.

Term	Definition
Insulin resistance	A condition in which cells become less responsive to insulin, requiring the pancreas to produce more to achieve normal glucose uptake. Precedes type 2 diabetes by years and is a driver of cardiovascular disease, dementia, and accelerated ageing.
MHT	Menopausal Hormone Therapy. The use of oestrogen (and typically progesterone in women with an intact uterus) to manage menopausal symptoms and reduce the health consequences of oestrogen deficiency. Modern formulations include transdermal oestradiol and micronised progesterone.
mTOR	Mechanistic target of rapamycin. A cellular sensor and regulator of growth and metabolism that, when chronically active, promotes cellular growth at the cost of repair and longevity. Inhibition of mTOR (by rapamycin, caloric restriction, or fasting) activates autophagy and extends lifespan in multiple model organisms.
NAD+	Nicotinamide adenine dinucleotide. A coenzyme central to energy metabolism, DNA repair, and activation of longevity-promoting sirtuins. Levels decline with age; NMN and NR are supplemental precursors used to raise NAD+ levels.

Term	Definition
PBS	Pharmaceutical Benefits Scheme. The Australian Government subsidy system for prescription medicines, covering eligible medications at significantly reduced cost for patients.
SASP	Senescence-Associated Secretory Phenotype. The cocktail of inflammatory cytokines and other signals secreted by senescent cells, which drives chronic inflammation and tissue damage in surrounding tissues.
Senolytics	Compounds that selectively clear senescent cells. Includes dasatinib plus quercetin (D+Q) and fisetin. Strong preclinical evidence; early human trials underway.
Sirtuins	A family of proteins (SIRT1–7) that regulate gene expression, DNA repair, metabolism, and cellular stress responses in ways that promote longevity. Activated by NAD+, caloric restriction, and exercise.
VO2 max	The maximum rate of oxygen consumption during maximal exercise. The single most powerful modifiable predictor of all-cause mortality; a direct measure of cardiorespiratory fitness.

Term	Definition
Zone 2 training	Aerobic exercise at approximately 60–70% of maximum heart rate, at which you can maintain a conversation but are clearly working. The primary driver of mitochondrial density and metabolic health adaptations.

Appendix E: Acknowledgements

This book was shaped by years of patients — first in pharmacy, then in medicine — who trusted me with their health and taught me, case by case, what it actually means to age well. Their stories, their questions, and their outcomes are the real evidence base for everything in these pages. I am grateful beyond what I can express in a single paragraph.

The scientists and clinicians whose work underpins this book are too numerous to list in full, but several deserve specific acknowledgement for the clarity and rigour they have brought to a field that is often obscured by commercial noise: the teams behind the NHANES cohort studies, the UK Biobank, the Dunedin Study, the American Gut Project, and the many dedicated researchers in epigenetics, exercise physiology, metabolic medicine, and geroscience whose work I have tried to represent accurately and honestly.

The Australian healthcare system — its GPs, specialists, allied health professionals, and the public health infrastructure that supports them — remains one of the great social achievements of this country.

My hope is that this book contributes, in some small way, to more Australians using it more effectively.

And finally: to everyone who picked up this book because they wanted to live better, not just longer. That distinction matters. This one was for you.